THE
ENZYME
FACTOR
2

ALSO BY HIROMI SHINYA MD

The Enzyme Factor

The Microbe Factor

The Enzyme Factor 2

THE ENZYME FACTOR 2

Reverse Aging
Stop Alzheimers
Prevent Diabetes
Improve Your Sex Life

Hiromi Shinya MD

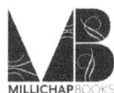

MILLICHAP BOOKS

Millichap Books, LLC

www.millichapbooks.com

Portions previously published in Japanese by Sunmark Press

First edition, second printing

Printed in the United States of America

Cover and interior design by Carl Brune

"Dr. Shinya's 7 Golden Keys for Good Health" was previously published in *The Enzyme Factor*.

ISBN 978-1-937462-23-9 (paperback)

ISBN 978-1-937462-25-3 (ebook)

Notice: This book is intended as a reference volume only, not as a medical manual. The information presented here is designed to help you make informed decisions about your health. It is not intended as a substitute for any treatment that may have been prescribed by your doctor, who is acquainted with your specific needs. If you suspect that you have a medical problem, we urge you to seek competent medical care.

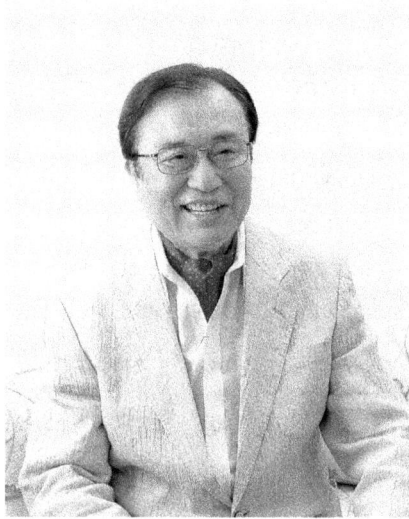

HIROMI SHINYA, M.D. is a world renowned gastroenterologist credited with the invention of the colonoscopy and the wire loop snare for removal of polyps without invasive surgery. Dr. Shinya was surgical professor at Albert Einstein Medical University and Director of Endoscopy at Beth Israel Hospital as well as an adviser for Maeda Hospital and Hanzomon Gastrointestinal Clinic in Japan.

In recent years Dr. Shinya has turned his attention and his inventive mind to the ways we can work with our body to strengthen and preserve our health. Using his many years of experience comparing the health of the colons of thousands to their diets and life styles, Dr. Shinya has made some exciting discoveries.

Dr Shinya's previous books, *The Enzyme Factor* and *The Microbe Factor* are international best sellers.

CONTENTS

CHAPTER 3
A lifestyle to elevate enzyme power

CHAPTER 4
Young mind, young body

Introduction

 Everybody wishes to be forever young, or at least to have the health and vitality of youth.

A man might brag, "I may not be as good as I once was, but I'm as good once as I ever was."

A woman might say, "I have aged and I don't really care."

Beneath such statements usually lies a wistful, unspoken desire to stay youthfully strong and beautiful, especially when we encounter a person our own age with the looks and vitality we seem to have lost in the last few years.

I was born in 1935 and I enjoy hearing people say I look younger than my age. Sometimes women, even young women, ask me what I do to preserve my skin. In this book I would like to reveal to you all my secrets for having smooth skin, vibrant energy, and a youthful zest for life. What I advocate is not cosmetic surgery, medications or wrinkle cremes. What I advocate costs little, can be safely adopted by anyone, and, most importantly, it works.

My rejuvenation method will engage both your mind and your body. My years of treating thousands of patients in my clinics in New York and Tokyo have shown me this truth about aging: No matter how good the method for your body, you cannot attain vibrant health and beauty if your mind is full of regrets and negative self-talk. On the other hand, no matter how positive your thoughts, your body cannot help aging if your lifestyle is unhealthy.

Why do people age? Why do some people of the same age look youthful while others look old? What exactly *is* aging?

My personal answer to this last question is that aging is the weakening of the body's enzyme power. Those of you who have read my books are already familiar with enzymes. We use the word enzyme as a collective term for vital protein catalysts inside the cells of living beings. Enzymes are necessary to all the processes and activities that maintain life in your body, such as synthesis, decomposition, digestion, elimination, and detoxification. It is my theory, based on years of clinical observations, that the aging process is accelerated by the body's declining enzyme power.

In this book, I will teach you how to defend against aging and declining enzyme power. I will suggest some guidelines for eating that I have seen work miracles to restore my patients' health and vitality. I will also suggest other lifestyle changes that will be simple for you to implement, if you are willing.

The eating guidelines I will share with you should not be considered a "diet" that you adopt temporarily and then abandon when you start looking and feeling better. What they are is a way of eating that discourages the oxidization of the body so that its enzyme power will not be compromised in its quality and quantity. I will show you exactly how to elevate and maximize your individual enzyme power.

Medically speaking, physical aging is a part of the cycle of our human life and it ultimately cannot be prevented. What is possible, however, is to prevent *unnecessary* aging. So much of the typical diet and lifestyle in our contemporary society, rather than promoting youth and vitality, actually causes premature aging. On the other hand, our medical science has progressed to the point where we know it is possible to rejuvenate a body which has prematurely aged back to the state appropriate for one's age. What is meant by 'appropriate for one's age?' Age appropriateness for the chronological age of the body is a number far younger today than what we thought possible just a few years ago.

Fifty really is the new forty and sixty the new fifty. The person you saw at the class reunion who looked younger than you and everyone else is exhibiting what I mean by age appropriateness. They haven't found some mythical fountain of youth, but they have maintained their health appropriate for their age. Their bodies are aging as the human body is ideally designed to age. Many others, perhaps most, have aged beyond their biological years for reasons of diet and lifestyle. When you wonder how a person can look so young for his/her age, you should instead see this youthful look as the possible, and now age-appropriate, health goal for all people—for *you*.

Mind and body are inseparable. One cannot attain youthfulness by taking good care of the body only, nor solely by thinking happy thoughts. As one hand washes the other, youthfulness comes from rejuvenating both body and mind. This book presents a mind/ body rejuvenation method to regain your innate, age-appropriate youthfulness, beauty and energy. I invite you to join me and begin what could very well be the best years of your life.

CHAPTER 1

The difference between younger-looking people and fast-aging people

Why new widows sometimes look rejuvenated

It is quite natural to want to stay young. Such a desire is probably instinctive. In many ways, nature can be our ally in seeking youthful vitality.

For instance, those of us in our sixties and seventies may, sadly, lose our mate. I have observed an interesting phenomenon when a woman loses her husband. Surprisingly, she looks rejuvenated! A female gets rejuvenated when she is divorced or widowed, while a male gets rejuvenated when he gets a new young lover or when he marries a young wife.

Of course this does not apply to everybody, nor is my opinion scientific, but it is based on my own observation. It doesn't mean the wife is glad to see the old guy go or that the husband is happy to be released to seek a younger bride.

The answer is in "mother nature," and has to do with hormones and endorphins. An interesting point here is that there is an element of love in both cases, and yet the contributing factor for rejuvenation is quite the opposite. Of course, there are women who have depleted their body enzymes from the stress of having lost their loved ones and as a result grow older. But men (like me) have noticed that women who have recently lost their husbands or who were recently divorced seem to get younger and more beautiful. Why does a woman who loses her loved one get younger? It is nature's way of helping her attract a new love. I realize you may feel offended by this statement, but please keep reading, because it makes sense from a biological point of view.

A female body is biologically designed to bear a child. A male body is designed to protect the female who will bear his child. It would make sense that it would be instinctive for women to want to be protected and for men to desire to protect them. It would also make sense for nature to maximize a woman's hormonal charm when she needs a man to protect her. In the same way, nature would maximize a man's charm when he finds a woman to protect. Thus, women who are separated by divorce or death from their mates become youthful and beautiful, while men who marry young wives of childbearing age become vigorous. We humans are part of the natural world, biologically programmed to maximize our survival and procreation.

When we fall in love at whatever age, we become young and beautiful. This is true for men and women alike. Falling in love is one of the most effective methods for rejuvenation since it elevates our enzyme power.

Luckily, we have the power to elevate our enzyme strength without losing a mate or finding a new romance. We can fall in love with a dream or have a strong purpose to be of service to someone else, to mankind, or to the planet. Only human beings are endowed with this power to improve our health and rejuvenate our energetic power by creating new purpose and meaning for our lives. Nature has endowed us with the simple purpose to live a long and healthy life and to stay youthful, but it may not be purpose enough to give us the necessary push. I would like you to think further about what you want to do with the extra years and extra energy you might gain by following the suggestions in this book. What would you do if you were young again? What goal or purpose would give you the strength of spirit and motivation of body to elevate your enzyme power? How might you fall in love with life today?

The reason I want to be youthful is that I have a strong motivation to see preventive medicine take root in our society. This is the purpose that inspires and excites me, and it keeps me vital. No matter how much I advocate habits of eating and living that promote wellness, however, nobody will listen to me if I do not practice in my own life what I advocate. It is very important for me to stay youthful in order to advocate how wonderful preventive medicine can be.

Spreading the good news about health, rejuvenation, and disease prevention is what inspires me. What is your inspiration? What would you do if you were younger, healthier, more energetic or more fit? Just having a goal or purpose clearly in front of you will help make it happen. I invite you to fall in love with life again. Your new vitality can help make the world a better place.

Skin reveals one's intestinal age

I can tell if a person has good intestinal features and good intestinal bacteria the moment he walks into my office and I look at his face. From experience, I know that people who look older than their chronological age have poor intestinal features. Facial features and intestinal features are closely related. Those with good facial features will have good intestinal features and those with poor intestinal features have poor facial features.

By facial features, I do not mean so-called "good looks." I mean the clinical conditions of the face, such as the condition of the person's skin, complexion, expression, or brightness of his or her eyes.

Most people think that as one grows older, the body gets weaker, the skin sags, the bones collapse, and that one will inevitably appear older. It is true that there is some physical decline as one gets older. Nobody is going to look at a man over 70 and mistake him for a teenager. Some of those over 70, however, are capable of looking like they are in their 50s or 60s. On the other hand, others might appear to be in their 80s or 90s. Our vague notion of age-appropriateness obviously cannot be trusted. In fact, there is no standard that states, "this is what appropriate aging looks like." The youthful look of our 50s may be the age appropriate look for some in their 70s.

How much decline must we accept as inevitable as we age? What is the difference between those who look younger and those who look older than their biological age? For most of us, we judge age by a person's skin. Firm and fresh-looking skin is a symbol of youth. Spots, wrinkles, and sagging flesh are signs of aging.

As it is with our skin tissues, so it is with our intestinal tissues. A person's intestinal features and his facial features are closely correlated. When intestinal features deteriorate, the most visible change one can observe is with the skin.

You may know that when you have constipation, you develop skin problems. Why does this happen?

The large and small intestines are the organs that digest and absorb foods. When your intestines are healthy, necessary nutrients are absorbed properly and waste from foods and toxins developed in the intestine are excreted. When one is constipated, however, toxins are not properly excreted, and as a result toxins in the intestine are passed to blood vessels through intestinal walls and circulate throughout the body. They are eventually excreted through sweat glands, causing damage to the skin. The relationship of constipation and skin disorders is a good example of the close relationship between your intestines and your skin.

Medical science has long known that most atopic dermatitis and allergens come from food and skin irritations, and that these conditions can be helped by strengthening the patient's immune functions. Those people with skin problems which are not caused by external factors usually have a problem stemming from their intestines. You could think of your skin as an external signal. What you see in the mirror will tell you a lot about how well things are functioning inside. People who appear older than their age probably have intestines that have aged prematurely.

The intestinal features of those who live beyond a century

When a person's intestinal features have aged more than his actual age, that person's lifespan will be shortened. The condition of someone's intestinal features is closely related to that person's lifespan.

As you read this, you may think that intestinal features deteriorate naturally as one ages, eventually becoming rigid by the time one dies. This is not the case. Of course there are people whose intestinal features deteriorate, leading to disease and eventually death. On the other hand, those people who die after having lived a long, healthy life have relatively good intestinal features.

I have examined many intestines of old people, including some centenarians. I have seen very poor intestinal features among some old people in their 80s, but I have never encountered poor intestinal features among people who are beyond 100 years old. The oldest person I have examined was 105 years of age and his intestine was soft and clean. It is interesting that there is hardly anyone over 90 who has poor intestinal features. To me, that means that the limit of the lifespan of most people with poor intestinal features is in the 80s, not the 90s. According to present day medicine, 120 years is the limit of a natural, healthy human life span.

My point is that people who make it past 100 years of age have relatively good intestinal features. People who don't have good intestinal features do not reach such an advanced age.

Perhaps you are one of those people who think, "It is okay. I'll keep eating, drinking and smoking whatever I feel like, because I don't want to live past my 80s." You may change your mind by the time you reach your late 70s. In fact, you may change your mind much earlier, if your lifestyle is making you feel and look like an old person. Whether we are talking about dietary habits or lifestyle, the damage to each person's health is unique. For example, I feel certain that ulcerative colitis or Crohn's disease is caused by excessive intake of dairy products, especially cow's milk, judging from my clinical experience examining thousands of patients and looking at their intestinal features as well as their dietary habits. Still, I don't know how much dairy is an "excessive" amount of dairy for you. I cannot tell the exact amount of dairy foods that would trigger the onset of the disease in any one person, because there is such great variation among individuals. Some may develop the disease from drinking a glass of milk once or twice a week, while some may never develop the disease even if they drink a quart of milk every day. The difference among individuals is enormous, yet it is certain that a diet and lifestyle that causes your body to use up large amounts of its stores of enzymes will eventually cause disease.

If a young person continues dietary habits that burden his intestines and consume his enzymes, it is certain he will be accelerating the aging of his intestines. It is possible for a 30-year-old man to have intestines of a person 70 years old. While one is young, a noticeable change may not be observed, due to the high recovery power of what I call the "miracle enzymes" (primary enzymes). After middle age, when the production of antacid enzymes, such as SOD (super oxide dismutase), slows down, the aging of the intestines is accelerated, spreading the aging process to all parts of the body. It is important to try to maintain healthy intestines to prevent such deterioration.

Diseases and aging stem from deteriorating intestinal features

The scientific study of the aging process has recently led to the proposal of various anti-aging methods. Quite a few of them are to treat only a few of the signs and symptoms of aging, such as treatments for the skin like Retin-A, or injections of hyaluronic acid or botox to smooth out wrinkles. Treating the signs of aging without addressing the causes of aging is not a true anti-aging method. The only true anti-aging method is to eliminate the causes of aging.

The biggest cause of aging is oxidization. Cells are damaged by oxidization and can no longer regenerate as normal cells. When oxidized substances invade your body, or when they are generated in your body, various types of antioxidants, especially enzymes, protect us by preventing our cells from damage. The larger the store of enzymes found in your body, the more difficult it is for the body to become oxidized.

The best way to maintain a large store of enzymes in your body is to follow dietary habits and a lifestyle that helps you maintain good intestinal features—intestines that are free of polyps and functioning well.

When your intestines must deal with a lot of decaying meat and other toxins, the internal culture of your intestinal features deteriorate. When there is a predominance of bad bacteria in your intestines, the intermediate bacteria in your gut get overwhelmed by the bad bacteria and they, too, go bad. Intermediate bacteria start out neither good nor bad, but become good or bad depending on the balance of the other bacteria in the gut, sort of like teenagers who are influenced by their peers. In other words, if the intestines contain a predominant amount of good bacteria, the intermediate bacteria will become good. If the intestines contain predominantly bad bacteria, the intermediate bacteria will go bad.

In addition, the good intestinal bacteria that are responsible for creating many of the enzymes we use every day will be overwhelmed by the bad bacteria generated by the toxins. Then, a large number of precious enzymes will be consumed to break down the toxins being generated inside our intestines, and this will weaken our ability for antioxidation. This shift from the dominance of good bacteria to the dominance of bad bacteria deteriorates the power of enzymes to replicate and impedes the immune system from operating at maximum efficiency.

The intestine is the largest immune organ in our body. When our intestine is invaded by a toxic substance, it reacts faster than any other organ and passes the information to the immune system. If the toxic substance is inside the intestine, it will cause diarrhea, your body's attempt to excrete toxins. If toxins invade other parts of the body, the immune system will send immune cells to eliminate the danger. White blood cells protect our bodies from invading viruses. There are natural killer cells which are known for their power to kill cancer cells and other lymphocyte cells such as T cells or B cells. Sixty to seventy percent of these cells are found inside our intestines. In other words, the intestines are the command center for the immune system of the entire body.

An intestine is a strange organ because it is not under the control of the brain. When someone suffers brain death, his heart and lungs stop functioning unless an artificial respirator is employed. His intestines, however, will continue to absorb nutrients and eliminate waste with no instruction from his brain. There are two types of autonomic nerves, sympathetic nerves and parasympathetic nerves, balancing our body's functions. The brain, the heart, and the lungs are under the control of the sympathetic nervous system. When we are tense or excited the sympathetic is the dominant nervous system. On the other hand, it is the parasympathetic nervous system that rules the stomach and intestines, and it is dominant while we are asleep or relaxed.

When you don't feel well, you will naturally want to lie down for rest. This urge to relax and sleep is nature's way of helping you to create conditions for the dominance of parasympathetic nerves, so that your immune system can work more efficiently. Even if your body is ready to follow directions from the intestines, however, if the intestine is fighting on two fronts, with toxins in the body and a diminished capacity to restore enzymes at the same time, these signals will be muddled, and the immune system cannot exercise its functions efficiently. This is why compromised intestinal health will lead to the compromised health of the entire body. Deterioration of your intestinal features reduces the number of enzymes available to your body and further compromises the production of new enzymes, thus further deteriorating your immune strength. Immune functions and enzyme power have reciprocal relations. One of the reasons why we become prone to diseases as we age is because of the deterioration of intestinal features.

The foods that facilitate aging & the foods that prevent aging

In order to maintain clean intestinal features, it is ideal to develop seven key health habits:

1. Proper diet
2. Good water
3. Proper elimination
4. Proper breathing
5. Moderate exercise
6. Good rest and sleep
7. Laughter and a sense of well-being

In my earlier books, I have outlined many specific ways in which to practice each of these essentials. I call them "essentials" because they work together, like ingredients in a recipe. If you leave out some of the ingredients, the recipe won't work as it is supposed to. I call this the *synergy effect*. Each one of these key habits works with every other one to maximize your health.

If you are at a loss as to where to start, I normally recommend that you start with changes in food and water.

We regenerate ourselves through metabolism by the food we eat. It is not an overstatement to say that the quality and extent of this regeneration depends on the quality of water and food we consume. Most people are concerned about the presumed nutritional value and calorie count of the food we buy and eat, but those qualities cannot prevent the aging process. If you wish to stay young, then it is necessary to adopt a diet that will keep your intestines young. You need to know what foods accelerate aging and what foods prevent aging. Let's start with foods that accelerate aging.

Oxidized foods are first on this list because oxidation creates free radicals in your body and free radicals damage cells and consume a large number of enzymes for detoxification. When you peel a potato or an apple, the surface turns brown after a while because the potato or apple is exposed to oxygen in the air. The longer a food is exposed to air, the more it gets oxidized. So, try to avoid foods which are brown or old. For cooking, avoid purchasing overly prepared foods such as pre-cut vegetables or meats. You should cut them up just before cooking to minimize oxidization. You should also minimize the use of foods which have been oxidized from the beginning, such as vegetable oils which are oxidized during the extraction process.

One entire group of foods that accelerate aging are *animal-based foods*. Meat is the biggest culprit. In Japan, people have come to believe that one needs meat for stamina and that one will not grow tall without it. It is true that the Japanese physique has become taller with the increase of meat consumption, but the reason for this is the accelerated speed of growth during the biological growth years. In other words, a larger physique is not the result of eating meat throughout life, but results from its consumption during the growth period. However, speedy growth is not necessarily healthy. Rapid growth implies rapid aging after a certain age.

Progeria syndrome is an intractable disease that causes the body to age quickly. It is a congenital defect of the genes, rather than the result of poor diet. People with this disease start aging in their childhood, because their aging speed is accelerated.

But a diet that regularly contains a lot of meat can also result in premature aging. The fat in animal meat cannot be dissolved at human body temperature; this fat therefore makes the blood thick. The temperature of popularly consumed meat ranges from 101-104 degrees Farenheit. Animal fat, which is liquid at such temperatures, begins to thicken in the human bloodstream which has a temperature of about 98.6. When blood does not flow smoothly, nutrients are not distributed to all parts of the cells. The adverse effect on cell metabolism promotes the aging process. It is important to remember that oxidized foods and animal foods, especially meat, are two major culprits that accelerate the aging process.

Plant-based foods lead to fine skin, animal-based foods to dry skin

The Japanese people used to be known for their fine skin. Now, however, their porcelain skin is becoming a glory of the past. Why have Japanese lost their lovely skin? This is attributable to their dietary changes. When I give a lecture, I sometimes let people touch my skin because I want them to feel the effect of my health method in preventing the aging of skin. My skin remains fresh and free from stains and spots, far from the tired-looking skin of many men in their 70s. People ask what I apply or where I go for treatments.

My "secret" is not a cream or a treatment. I simply follow the health method I have been recommending to my patients for years. I drink good water and eat so as to have healthy intestines. The reason why Japanese used to have smooth skin was the Japanese diet. The reason why many Japanese have lost their beautiful skin is the loss of the Japanese dietary culture.

What was the Japanese diet? It was a plant-based diet with whole grains as the main staple. A traditional Japanese meal used to consist of brown rice, soybean soup, cooked vegetables and sea weeds and some fish. During the fast economic growth after World War II, people lost interest in such fare, and their diet was taken over by more gorgeous-looking steaks, hamburgers and other meats.

A diet consisting of mostly plant-based foods with whole grains as the main dish is ideal not only for Japanese but for everyone. Such a notion came to the fore after the McGovern report was published in the U.S. in 1977. The report stated that the most ideal meal is the Japanese diet prior to the Genroku Era. The Japanese diet before the Genroku Era was mostly unrefined rice. Unrefined brown rice contains carbohydrates, dietary fibers, vitamins, minerals, and enzymes. Such good quality carbohydrates are digested and absorbed very efficiently, without generating toxins which are often produced when digesting proteins and fats. Furthermore, with such a sufficient amount of dietary fibers, waste and toxins are eliminated without constipation. The germ or outer husk of the grain is lost when refining rice. There is a nutrient called phytic acid in the germ that promotes the elimination of the pesticide residues from the many pesticides that are now employed in growing grains and vegetables. Brown rice that has not been over-refined helps eliminate this pesticide residue.

The real value of the Japanese diet is not limited to its healthy qualities. The "traditional diet" which the Japanese have adopted for hundreds of years is most suitable to them. The ability to digest foods varies among groups of people. Each group has evolved the enzymes, bacteria, and intestinal length to digest foods that are a part of their traditional diet. There is a vast difference in their ability to assimilate and digest animal-based proteins and fats between Europeans who have been eating animals for thousands of years and the Japanese who have been following plant-based diets. At the same time, the Western diet is unhealthy even for ethnic Europeans who have grown used to eating and digesting meat. Even they suffer less from the effects of premature aging and have healthier skin when they follow a diet that emphasizes vegetables, fruits, legumes and whole grains.

Atkins diet deteriorates intestinal features

Some say that carbohydrates lead to weight gain and therefore one should minimize the intake of carbohydrates in order to lose weight. If you stick with a diet with minimal carbohydrates for six months or more, however, your intestinal features will deteriorate dramatically.

One low-carbohydrate diet called the Atkins diet has been intermittently popular in the U.S. for years. I have examined the intestines of many people who have followed this diet and I found that all of these patients suffered from poor intestinal features. The intestines of those who had followed this diet for more than a year were invariably hard, with narrowed cavities. Some had even developed diverticulitis.

Dr. Atkins' office was in my neighborhood. I knew him personally and I challenged him on this diet, telling him that any diet with as few carbohydrates as his would lead to poor intestinal features and endanger his patients' health. I told him I was examining people who had been on the diet and this was what I was finding. He denied the truth of my findings, but, sadly, died himself soon after our conversation in April, 2003. He was only 72.

The reason one loses weight by eliminating carbohydrates is the same reason a diabetic patient suddenly loses weight. In our body, the intake of carbohydrates elevates the glucose level and stimulates the pancreas to generate insulin. Insulin is a hormone that induces blood sugar to be sent to the inside of our cells. Diabetes is a disease with poor or compromised insulin secretion from the pancreas. Without insulin, glucose in the blood cannot enter or be fed to cells, causing a state of starvation. Body fat is then broken down to generate the needed energy.

The problem is that a strong oxidized substance called *ketone* is generated during this sort of fat metabolism. Ketone is usually excreted through urine, sweat and breath, but when there is a very large amount of ketone in the body it exceeds one's ability to excrete it in the usual way. When this happens your blood, which should be mildly alkaline, turns acidic. In extreme cases ketoacidosis develops that can threaten your life.

Even if you do not reach such an extreme state of ketoacidosis, you can easily see why such a dangerous diet is not good for your body. The Atkins diet dangerously turns the body acidic by its excessive intake of protein. This kind of diet damages fat, muscles and organs. Among those following the Atkins diet, many suffer from migraines, muscle spasms, and diarrhea. This is the body's way of signaling that something is wrong. The body is sending you an SOS for help.

Another problem resulting from the Atkins diet is that it does not provide any limit to the amount of animal-based protein and fat. The reason one does not gain weight from a large amount of protein is that excess protein is not absorbed by the body and is excreted. It is a mistake to think that one can eat all the protein one wants if it does not cause weight gain. The excess protein is not simply excreted. It is broken down into amino acids, and these amino acids are further broken down to excrete as urine.

Needless to say, a large number of enzymes are used for this work of breaking down the excess protein. Furthermore, in breaking down amino acid, various types of hazardous acids, such as urea, uric acid, and pyruvic acid are generated. This turns the blood acidic. This oxidized blood must be neutralized with the help of calcium, so calcium is then pulled out of bones and teeth. Meanwhile, if you are not consuming enough water, your urine gets very dense, damaging the kidneys.

In addition, protein does not go into making feces. Although the Atkins diet does recommend the consumption of certain vegetables, an adequate amount of roughage is not generated without the consumption of carbohydrates with good quality fibers. When an inadequate amount of feces is generated, the flow in the stomach and intestines is compromised, leading to deteriorated intestinal features.

Also, the Atkins diet does not limit the amount of fat consumption. When you eat too much fat, the blood gets thick, inhibiting the distribution of oxygen and nutrients to the entire body (again, too much fat in the bloodstream thickens the blood because fat begins to coagulate at body temperature). Without the distribution by the blood of an adequate amount of nutrients and oxygen, the mitochondria in the cells cannot function, thus inhibiting metabolism in the cells. Needless to say, too much of this causes unnecessary aging.

Losing weight does not necessarily lead to good health. It is meaningless to attain a slim body if your organs are compromised. In order to lose weight and stay healthy, it is necessary to have a diet of good quality carbohydrates such as brown rice and other unrefined grains and, of course, good water. You may not achieve the instantaneous loss of weight that you might on a diet like the Atkins, but you lose weight in a healthy fashion without burdening the body, weight you are less likely to regain immediately. This kind of high fiber diet also brings the added benefit of cleaning your stomach and intestines.

Difference between visceral fat type and subcutaneous fat type

There are increasingly older men and women who are dieting seriously. One of the reasons is an epidemic of what is popularly called "metabolic syndrome." Briefly stated, metabolic syndrome implies the condition of a person who has visceral fat with elevated blood sugar, high blood pressure and high cholesterol, and who is therefore prone to atherosclerosis. The label of metabolic syndrome was announced as a diagnostic standard by the World Health Organization (WHO) in 1998. You probably have metabolic syndrome if you have a waist line at your navel that exceeds 33.5" for men and 35.4" for women combined with any two of the following:

1. Fasting blood sugar level of 110mg/dl or more
2. Blood pressure of 130/85 (either or both) or more
3. HDL (over 150mg/dl). LDL (less than 40mg/dl) (either or both)

The most noticeable characteristic of metabolic syndrome is that it is associated with visceral fat type, and not subcutaneous fat type. When caloric intake exceeds the amount of calories spent, the excess calories are stored as fat. There are two types of fat; subcutaneous fat, which is located right under the skin; and visceral fat, which is located around internal organs. The characteristic of subcutaneous fat is that the area where the fat is attached is soft and one can pinch the area. The kind of fat that is easy to grab is often found among middle-aged women. On the other hand, visceral fat is located between abdominal muscles and organs, typically characterized by a portly belly.

The reason why a body of the visceral fat type is the target of this syndrome is because a majority of hyperlipidemia patients are visceral-fat-type people. Each of these conditions—high blood sugar, high blood pressure and high HDL cholesterol/low LDL cholesterol—poses a high risk for health, and when in combination, can lead to a very high risk state, such as arterial sclerosis. From my experience examining the intestines of both types, I have seen the difference in terms of their intestinal features between visceral-fat-types and subcutaneous-fat-types. It does not apply to all, but many subcutaneous-fat-type people have soft and good looking intestines. In other words, quite a number of subcutaneous-fat-type people are healthy. On the other hand, most visceral-fat-type people have poor intestinal features. The health of visceral-fat-types is definitely at risk. The intestines of people with visceral fat are thick and hard, and they often have diverticula. Some people don't look fat but have visceral fat; I can tell this from a heavy feeling when I am operating a colonoscope in the intestine. The effects of visceral fat and subcutaneous fat are quite different.

Excessive intake of animal-based food leads to visceral fat

Why do some people develop visceral fat while some develop subcutaneous fat?

In today's medicine, both are deemed to be the result of excess calorie intake and lack of exercise. The cause for the difference is said to be unknown. Thus, in order to cure metabolic syndrome, the general recommendation is for dietary restriction of calorie intake and regular exercise. Since visceral fat is likely a source of energy when muscles are used, it is believed that men who generally have more muscles than women are likely to develop visceral fat. This is, however, a relative comparison, and visceral fat is found in many women. Furthermore, those men with visceral fat, although they are not labeled as having metabolic syndrome, generally have little muscle and do not get much exercise. Thus, it is my opinion that it is not necessarily true to state that visceral fat is stored in people with big muscles. So, what is the cause of visceral fat?

Both visceral fat and subcutaneous fat come from food we consume.

I made a comparison of the diets of those with a large amount of visceral fat and those with a large amount of subcutaneous fat. I found a remarkable difference between them. The amount of animal-based fat was at least partially the answer. Many of those with visceral fat were big consumers of fatty meat and fatty dairy products. The subcutaneous-fat-type people tended to eat foods using plant-based oil, rather than animal fats. It interested me that those people who consumed large amounts of fat from animal and dairy foods developed more visceral fat than their counterparts of equal weight with subcutaneous fat. My hypotheses is that fat from animals whose body temperature is higher than that of humans may contribute to visceral fat stores. The individuals with a heavy weight who did not have visceral fat were more likely to eat fish than meat or dairy.

People store excess calories as subcutaneous fat as a biological preparation for starvation. When food and water might not be accessible, fat stored in the body supplies energy and water. You may be surprised to learn that water is stored in fat, but it is not hard to comprehend when you know that the humps of a camel store fat and those humps supply water to the body of the camels when needed. If subcutaneous fat is the supply source of water and energy, however, what is the purpose of visceral fat? I believe that the body stores visceral fat as a "buffer" to protect our intestines that have been damaged by excess consumption of animal-based fat. People who consume a large amount of fat and protein from animal-based food get fewer enzymes from food intake, so they use up a large amount of their base of enzymes for digestion and breaking down toxins generated inside the body.

The amount of what I call miracle enzymes or base enzymes in their body tends to be low. At the same time, deterioration inside their intestines invites an increasing number of inflammatory microorganisms. The mucous membranes of their intestines will generate a large amount of histamine and free radicals. What ensues is an allergic reaction to irritants. In other words, visceral fat is formed to protect intestines which, due to the excess intake of animal-based protein and fat, have been hardened, narrowed and shortened, and so are hyper-reactive to external irritation.

The mechanism of visceral fat formation has not been proven. What I have stated is my medical hypothesis. However, based on my clinical experience with thousands of patients, taking their dietary histories and scoping their intestines over the course of 30 years, I can say unequivocally that people with heavy consumption of animal-based fat tend to have visceral fat. I urge researchers to identify the mechanism of visceral fat formation.

Fatty liver, alcohol and the overfed goose

I will cite alcohol as another culprit that causes visceral fat. It is well known that excessive alcohol intake will turn a healthy liver into a fatty liver. A fatty liver implies excess fat storage in the liver.

The liver is an important organ which stores the nutrients absorbed by the intestines and sends these nutrients to all parts of the body. For example, protein is broken down as amino acid in the intestines and is sent to the liver. The liver, in turn, re-synthesizes the amino acid as protein suitable for absorption in the human body. Similarly, the fat, which is broken down and absorbed as fatty acid in the intestines, is changed to cholesterol, phosphatide, serum triglyceride and so forth, and these are sent to all parts of the body. Even a healthy liver has 3-5% fat at all times.

When the function of the liver deteriorates, or when the liver is fed with an excessive amount of nutrients from overeating, the balance between the supply and demand is compromised, and excess fat accumulates in the liver. Generally speaking, when the amount of fat in a liver exceeds 30%, it is diagnosed as a *fatty liver*. The *fois gras* you might see on a restaurant menu is nothing more than the fatty liver of an overfed duck or goose.

Another type of fatty liver develops from the excess intake of alcohol. The mechanism to develop a fatty liver from alcohol is a little different from the mechanism that results from overeating. Alcohol is absorbed in the intestines, but 20% of the alcohol consumed has already been absorbed by the stomach. The alcohol sent from the stomach to the liver is first broken down into the very toxic substance, acetaldehyde. This hazardous acetaldehyde is further broken down by enzymes into acetic acid before eventually breaking down into water and carbon dioxide and excreted. This breakdown process doesn't proceed in a single flow. Instead, the alcohol that has not yet been broken down and the acetaldehyde circulate through the body over and over until they are completely broken down.

While the alcohol is circulating, the body is in a drunken state. When acetaldehyde is not broken down completely and remains in the body, the person suffers nausea, headache and other aches and pains, *aka* a hangover.

There are many stages needed to break down alcohol in the system, and at each stage enzymes are consumed. Furthermore, a large amount of active oxygen is generated at each stage of breakdown and more enzymes are consumed to detoxify the excess of active oxygen. This process is possible if there are enough enzymes in the body. People who have been heavy drinkers generally lack a sufficient amount of enzymes, and they are thus unable to repair the damage done by the overabundance of active oxygen. As a result, excessive active oxygen destroys liver cells, causing gaps in the liver. The liver, in order to fill such a gap, will use fat found nearby. Alcoholic fatty liver is the result of toxins generated during the repetitive breakdown of alcohol , which in turn creates cell damage and the body's attempt to plug the resultant holes in the liver, using fat.

Trading youth for meat and drink

I have little doubt that an excessive intake of animal-based foods and alcohol will make you old before your time. This is because a diet heavy in animal fat coupled with excessive drinking leads to increasing visceral fat, which accelerates the aging process.

At present, a well balanced, low-calorie diet in addition to exercise are generally recommended for those diagnosed with metabolic syndrome. It is true that exercise will reduce visceral fat, but as to the diet, a little more specific advice is needed. What exactly is a well balanced, nutritional diet, based on clinical research? The effect of various foods on the body should be studied, and patients should be advised to avoid those foods which are likely to turn to visceral fat.

Much present day nutritional science simply ignores the difference between animal protein and vegetable protein. According to my clinical data, however, these have completely different effects on our body.

Thus, I advise my patients with high amounts of visceral fat to reduce the intake of animal-based foods as the first step. My recommendation is to limit meat consumption to once or twice a month, to eat fish about twice a week since its fat is different from other animal fat, and to try to get protein from plant-based foods such as legumes. In order to improve my patients' intestinal features, I recommend a meal of grains (brown rice mixed with other grains) as a staple food, along with vegetables, sea vegetables, and fruits. I also recommend an adequate amount of water to facilitate the flow of blood and lymph. By such means, visceral fats are reduced and intestinal features show remarkable improvements in 3-6 months.

Our bodies are often wiser than we are. They are always trying to improve and balance our health, aiming at optimal health. Our desire to eat more and to drink more result in the waste of our enzymes, placing a burden on our organs. A little bit of self-discipline to restrain our urges for alcohol and animal-based foods will pay huge dividends in improved health.

I am Japanese, but I do not agree with the Japanese saying that "Sake is the best medicine," nor do I believe in the biblical injunction to "Take a little wine for the stomach." Alcohol does the body absolutely no good.

I don't drink at all, but I had an experience of collapsing from a drink that contained alcohol, which I drank by mistake. It was a hot day and when I returned to the clubhouse after a round of golf I was quite dehydrated. At the bar, my wife ordered a piña colada and I ordered a virgin piña colada. The bartender must have switched the drinks and I had a sip of the one with alcohol. Even though I detected the taste of alcohol and did not drink the whole drink, it was too late. My blood pressure and my heart rate started going up in only a few minutes. Since the amount I drank was small, my blood pressure and heart rate returned to normal after a while, and nothing serious happened.

I may be an extreme case, but keep in mind that to some people alcohol is quite toxic. More than 50% of Japanese are said not to have the enzymes to break down alcohol, and yet there are many who can consume alcohol. This is because enzymes tend to be placed where they are often used. Those who could not initially drink much can become heavy drinkers if they continue the practice. This is because the body knows the danger and places enzymes for detoxification. But the development of the ability to break down alcohol is not necessarily good because it comes at the expense of the consumption of a large number of the body's enzymes.

Drinks may have the merit of releasing stress or acting as a social lubricant for human relationships, but there are better ways to achieve these goals. It is important to realize that drinking is overtaxing your body.

Women are especially vulnerable to the negative effects of drinking. For one thing, they are also more prone to becoming addicted to alcohol. Many women get drunk more easily after menstruation. This is because they have higher amounts of estrogen. In addition, it takes longer for women to metabolize alcohol. More time for alcohol metabolism implies a longer time for toxins to stay inside the body, increasing risk.

Please realize, ladies, that you are paying for the drink that may be fun at the time with your youth. Those who make efforts not to waste enzymes may enjoy a drink once in a while, but if you make a habit of drinking, telling yourself the amount is tolerable, after years of such a habit, you may be the victim of premature aging or a fatty liver.

The more you desire to stay young, the younger you look

The difference between men and women who look younger and those who look older is also reflected in their intestinal features. Those with clean intestinal features have youthful skin, and those with poor intestinal features have aged skin and look older than their actual years.

If you wish to stay young, it is important for you to follow a diet and a lifestyle to improve your stomach and intestinal features. And it is never too late to start turning back the clock. With improved stomach and intestinal features it is certain that you will become healthier and you are likely to look younger as a result.

Sometimes, however, there are people who look youthful without any effort to improve their stomach and intestines. Similarly, some of the people who adhere to a good diet and lifestyle look more youthful, while some don't. What is the difference between those who look younger and those who don't?

I have learned the answer to this mystery through many years of examining and getting to know my patients. Those who look particularly youthful have a strong desire to be youthful. In other words, their mindset is different. I will elaborate this point later. The effect of the mind on the body is far greater than medical science has realized in the past.

I have stated in my previous books that drive and positive motivation can conquer diseases. Similarly, the degree of your youthful appearance varies with the strength of your desire.

Among actresses and famous people, you will find many who look younger than their biological age. They are not necessarily following a diet to improve their stomach and intestines. Their youthful looks come from their strong desire to be young and beautiful. Their look may not be backed by their health, but it is plausible that their strong desire has a good effect on their bodies. As proof of this, there are quite a few retired actresses and presidents who have aged rapidly; this is because of their diminished desire. If their youthfulness were backed with their health, they wouldn't age so fast. Your strong intentions do matter. The best approach is to practice diet and lifestyle which are good for your intestines, but also to cultivate a strong desire to be youthful.

For someone like myself who practices preventive medicine, I have to live what I teach or no one will listen. It is important for me to be and to look healthy and youthful. I advocate methods I have developed to live a life free from disease. The more meaningful it is to live such a life—the stronger the desire one has—the healthier one can stay.

CHAPTER 2

How to Regain Youthful Health and Beauty

Water—overlooked by many anti-aging methods

We appreciate fresh, smooth and youthful skin just as we appreciate fresh juicy fruits. High fluid content is an indication that cells are young and healthy. On average, 60–70% of a human body is made of fluid. The younger a person is, the more likely he or she will be on the high end of that percentage, because the body tends to lose fluid as we age. Fluid in a baby is 70-80% of the body weight, 60–70% for a grown up, declining to 50-60% for a senior. This is an indication of the close relationship between aging and cells that are plump with fluid—or not. The stomachs and intestines of babies are very beautiful, smooth, and finely textured, like their skin. The amount of fluid in the skin of a baby can be as high as 88%. By the time we are 20, that fluid may drop to 68%. At the age of 60 the amount of fluid in the body decreases to perhaps 40%.

The reason why the hyaluronan growth hormone is becoming popular for anti-aging regimens is because hyaluronan has the power to elevate the moisture content in the skin. Hyaluronan is a moisture-retention agent. The growth hormone starts declining at approximately 15 years of age. Many anti-aging methods attempt to rejuvenate the skin by artificially supplementing this growth hormone. In my opinion this is not a good idea, as such a method may have risks.

There are many things about the way our body functions that we do not fully understand. For example, the hormones we secrete in our teens regulate our growth and turn on puberty. We need lots of growth hormones during this important developmental time. The secretion of growth hormones reaches a peak in our teens. We continue to secrete some growth hormones after we reach adulthood, because growth hormones are required for metabolism and immune functions, but the amount we need is far less than when we were teens.

Is it proper to supplement growth hormones to keep the skin

soft and smooth after the person has reached adulthood, ignoring the natural rhythms of nature and the body? The effect of growth hormones on skin has been proven, but its effect on other parts of our body over a long period should be researched before we use growth hormones for such a purpose. Hormones are vital for our existence, and yet the amount we need is very small. It is so easy to upset the delicate hormonal balance in the body that I don't think such an artificial supplement is the best choice for our health.

What is necessary to attain a healthy and youthful body should not be artificially supplemented. Instead, we should work to create the conditions inside our body that will bring out the body's innate homeostatic mechanism and natural healing power. In order to attain such conditions, we should employ the natural means of good food, good water, proper elimination, adequate sleep, deep breathing, physical exercise and a positive mental state.

Many so-called anti-aging methods are oblivious to the one most important natural way to good health and beauty—*drinking good water!* Good water in adequate supply is your most powerful beauty secret. One cannot expect to have the dewy skin of youth using moisture retentive substances or hormones while dehydrating the body with an inadequate supply of good water. Water has a greater impact on the health and function of your body than food. It is a mistake to think of increasing moisture retention by using hormone therapy while forgetting to supply your body with the right kind of water.

Why the first sign of aging is detected on skin

Water is found in all parts of the body. Even dry looking nails contain about 15% water. We need water to carry necessary nutrients and excrete waste, of course, but its role is not limited to those functions. Enzymes cannot function without water. In order to get full enzyme power, a large amount of water is necessary. This is because an adequate supply of water regulates the flow in the stomach and intestines as well as the elimination of toxins, and it thus regulates the balance of bacteria inside cells in the intestines, contributing to the generation of more enzymes.

Water plays a vital role in the immune system. For example, if the body is dehydrated, the trachea is not moist, and immune cells cannot function properly. Their ability to ward off fungus and viruses diminishes. The inadequately hydrated body becomes prone to colds, coughing, bronchitis, or pneumonia.

This is not limited to mucous membranes such as the trachea. Skin which is constantly exposed to air could become dry and less resistant to various bacteria, leading to skin troubles such as dermatitis. So-called sensitive skin that reacts with rashes and other skin problems from little irritation is skin with inadequate moisture in the cuticle layer. The skin, which is so vital as a protective covering for the body, can only protect us when its cells have the moisture they need.

Water is vital for all the internal organs as well. The body's innate intelligence understands that there may not be an adequate water supply all the time. Thus, wired into the body is its own order of priority for the supply of water to our vital organs.

The first priority goes to the brain. The brain is a mass of nerve cells, 85% of which is comprised of water. The brain processes information gathered through nerves in all parts of the body and issues whatever instructions are necessary to keep everything functioning. The reason why a brain contains such a large percentage of water is because water acts as a medium for carrying information. There are minute channels inside nerve cells, and nerve transmitter substances produced in the brain are conveyed through these channels to peripheral nerves. Thus, a shortage of water in the brain will result in a failure to convey information to and instructions from the brain. In short, the brain is unable to handle information vital to the body's survival. If the shortage of water is slight, you may just suffer a headache, but if the shortage of water is serious, it can lead to symptoms such as a disturbance of consciousness or a disorder of memory. With an extreme shortage of water, like that seen in heat stroke, your survival will be at risk.

The body's water priority after the brain is the lungs, followed by the endocrine system, including the liver and kidneys. Muscles and bones rank low in priority. The last priority is the skin. This is why the signs of aging are observed mostly on the skin.

Lack of water intake can lead to cancer

An average size adult requires about 1.5-2 liters of water. If you drink only 1 liter a day, your body will suffer the effects of a water shortage of 30-50%. The shortage is not evenly shared by all organs and cells because the body will prioritize the distribution of water to the organs according to their importance for life. In other words, a third to a half of your skin cells, which rank low in priority, will not get any water. Dehydration in an organ such as the brain or the heart would threaten your life. Dehydration in your skin will make it less elastic, but this will not cause death. Thus, when there is a shortage of water, the body will adjust the flow of blood to peripheral blood vessels and prioritize the flow to the most vital parts.

At the same time, the body's ability to prioritize the distribution of water ensures that your blood pressure will be maintained at an adequate level, so as not to compromise the supply of nutrients and oxygen to the cells and the elimination of waste from cells. A human body can tolerate a deprivation of food and water to a certain degree and those cells deprived of water will not die immediately. If such a condition continues, however, cells will lose the ability for normal metabolism and normal functions.

In those cells that lack water to eliminate toxins, enzymes cannot function properly and there is a greater danger for a mutation of genes, which leads to cancer. Some may not believe that a shortage of water intake may lead to an onset of cancer, but this is the truth.

A 23 -year-old Japanese man visited my clinic in New York for a consultation. He was suffering from dysphagia (trouble swallowing) since he had cancer between his esophagus and stomach. Suspecting that a lack of water might be part of the problem, I asked how much water he drinks in a day. His reply was that he drinks more than average people. His skin was rough, his circulation was poor, and also an endoscopic observation indicated a shortage of water. Upon further questioning, I found that he was not drinking any water at all. He was drinking carbonated soda pop containing a great deal of caffeine, which deprives the body of water. He was consuming 7-8 bottles a day.

Water is a fluid, but not all fluids are water. I'll elaborate on this later, but it is important to realize that what our body needs is not just any fluid. It needs water. I came to know the importance of consuming an adequate amount of water through my research on dietary habits and diseases. The majority of my cancer patients have not had adequate water.

When I operate on a cancer patient, I recommend seven specific health habits to prevent a recurrence of the cancer, especially emphasizing that they need to drink a large amount of water. 1.5-2 liters (or 1.5-2 quarts) a day is adequate for a healthy person, but I recommend 2-3 liters (or 2-3 quarts) of water as long as there are no problems with the kidneys. I believe one of the reasons why the cancer recurrence rate among my patients is low is attributable to such guidance.

There are many alternatives to Western medicine, which involves mostly surgery and pharmaceuticals. The enzyme therapy I advocate is one of them. The "water cure," which advocates an adequate supply of water to cure diseases, is another. An Iranian medical doctor, Dr. Batmanghekudj, researched the importance of the role of water and stated that most modern day diseases stem from compromised metabolism due to a chronic shortage of water in the cells. His book has been read widely, and many people suffering from chronic diseases have been cured. I read his book and I agree with his theory that shortage of water in the cells is the cause of many problems, although I cannot agree that *all* diseases are caused by a shortage of water. My recommendation is to follow a regimen consisting of eating the right food, drinking enough good water, regular elimination, breathing, adequate exercise, good sleep, and relaxation for a peaceful mind. Health is maintained through the interaction of all these practices. It may even be dangerous to believe that *only* food or *only* water alone can cure disease. No matter how well balanced a person's diet is, the effect is not adequate to restore and maintain health unless enough water is consumed. In fact, it is important to practice all seven health methods.

Your body needs water at all times

When do you drink water? If your answer is, "When I am thirsty," your body is probably quite dehydrated. Thirst is the *last* signal from the body warning of a shortage of water. What is the first signal? It may well be elevated blood pressure or dry skin.

The first impact of water shortage in the body is on the blood and lymph system. The major role of blood is to carry oxygen and energy to cells, while lymph carries away old cells and waste. You can think of the blood and lymph systems as the waterworks and sewage systems for the body. Blood is comprised of blood cells and blood plasma. Plasma, which comprises 60% of the blood, is 90% water. Lymph is found in lymph vessels after plasma from blood capillaries flows into lymph channels. The lymph is also comprised of 90% water.

When a body does not have enough water, there is not enough water in blood and lymph. The result is thick blood. This is the first signal of too little water in the body. When blood is thick, its flow is compromised. The body tries to ensure the flow to vital organs by raising blood pressure, increasing one's heart rate or shutting down capillary blood vessels. The first sign or warning of a shortage of water is declining skin tone. Perhaps you have noticed how skin becomes rejuvenated with massage. This is because the stimulation of the massage increases the flow of blood into capillary vessels. Changes in blood pressure or skin tone should be seen as signals warning of a chronic shortage of water.

There are, however, many other ways the body sends warning signals. For example, when I speak for a long time in a lecture, I develop hoarseness, a sign of water shortage. I make a habit of drinking enough water, but during a lecture I lose a large amount of water in a short span of time from breathing and sweating. The lungs and trachea are constantly in need of water and therefore their water supplies are prioritized, but when a large amount of water is consumed, dehydration develops rapidly. Those people who often give speeches or sing should drink about a liter (quart) of water before the performance. There are increasing numbers of people suffering from dry eyes due to the use of computers. Rather than treating this as a problem with the eyes, my suggestion is to drink 2-3 glasses of water and close your eyes for a while. This is a safer and much more effective method than using eye drops. The best cure, however, is prevention: drink plenty of water regularly so that the body has an adequate water supply at all times.

Perhaps you have experienced cramps in your legs at night. This is also a sign of water shortage in your body. A cramp is caused by a contraction in the calf muscle. The cause for such a contraction is an imbalance of minerals from water shortage in the blood. This is also true with cramps that happen after vigorous exercise, such as swimming or soccer. During sleep, one is prone to dehydration because the body is deprived of water for several hours. One is also prone to sweat at night to regulate the body. The average adult sweats the equivalent of one glass of water during a night's sleep. Drinking water right before going to bed, however, should be avoided because of the danger of back-flow from stomach to esophagus. I suggest that you drink water about 2 hours before retiring and pass excess water through urination prior to retiring.

Those suffering from allergies or atopic dermatitis should drink water

Basic heath examinations always include a urine analysis. Urine excreted from the body contains many clues about an individual's health. The urine that is passed first in the morning is best for a urine analysis because it is the least diluted. The patient has not been drinking water for eight hours and his urine therefore has the least amount of water and is the most dense. The color indicates the urine's density. The urine of a healthy person who consumes a healthy amount of water is clear with just a tint of yellow. Healthy urine in the morning is a little darker.

The color of urine gets darker as water in the body decreases, so those with dark colored urine in the morning should increase their water consumption. Older people whose water retention rate is low and babies who require a large amount of water are prone to becoming dehydrated. It is especially important for the elderly and very young to supplement water often. Innate systems in the adult body regulate water by shrinking vessels or decreasing the volume of urine. The color and density of the urine changes accordingly. The bodies of babies, however, have not developed enough to regulate the body fluid in this way. That is why it is important to pay attention to their fluid intake in order to keep them adequately hydrated. Dehydration might be the cause when a baby keeps crying after a full meal. It is especially important to pay attention to a baby's hydration when the infant is fed with baby formula, since formulas are manufactured with ingredients resembling breast milk, though the base material is usually cow's milk. Animal-based foods tend to make the body acidic and as a result prone to dehydration. Babies with weak stomachs and intestines are in danger of developing intestinal inflammation or increased histamine secretion from the stress of dehydration.

Speaking of histamine, I'd like to touch on the adverse effect of dehydration on allergies. Histamine is a substance that sends a signal to the immune system when an allergen invades the body. In other words, histamine is released as a signal to purge an invading organism. When histamine is released in excess, it causes various types of allergic reactions, such as a runny nose, inflammation, itchiness, edema, and pain. The same is basically true with atopic dermatitis and asthma. Those who suffer from allergic symptoms have elevated histamine releases. Histamine is useful for the body as a transmitter for the immune system, as long as it is not released in excess. Why, you might ask, is histamine released in excess? We don't have an answer at present. Since heredity is observed in allergies, researchers are trying to see if this is a genetic issue, but so far it has not been determined to be so.

Interestingly, experiments with animals have confirmed that with an increase in water supply to the body, the production of histamine is reduced. Dr. Batmanghekudj, who advocates "Water Care," reported that when his patients suffering from allergies increased their water consumption, the symptoms were amazingly reduced. I don't know exactly why the increase in water consumption leads to reduced histamine production, but I suspect that an adequate amount of water in the cells acts as a kind of "barrier" of mucosa, so that cells start functioning properly to suppress the adverse reaction to allergic substances.

The brain after a night of drinking is surprisingly shrunken

If you have ever used alcohol, you have no doubt experienced a burning thirst in the morning after a night of heavy drinking. This happens because the body is extremely dehydrated.

Alcohol deprives the body of water in various ways. The first is on account of the diuretic property of alcohol. Heavy beer drinkers can chug their beers because the water lost as urine is far greater than the water they take in from the beer. Water in the body also gets used to neutralize and eliminate toxins generated during the course of alcohol breakdown. The body wants to dispose of toxins as soon as possible, so the volume of urine increases for this purpose, depleting the water in the body. Furthermore, when alcohol is consumed, the amount of water evaporating from the membrane of the nose increases due to the alcohol in the breath. Alcohol makes water more volatile. At the same time, immediately after consuming alcohol, blood vessels expand, speeding blood flow, and the heart rate increases, followed by a high respiratory rate. With increased respiratory rates, water is lost from the trachea more rapidly. With increased blood circulation the body temperature rises and the amount of sweat to regulate the body temperature increases also. In this way, a large amount of water in the body is lost, causing dehydration.

When dehydration continues, a rebound in the blood flow occurs. In other words, in order to protect the body from the rapidly advancing dehydration state, blood vessels shrink to limit the blood flow. When blood vessels contract, restricting the blood flow to capillary vessels, a large number of cells become inefficient. In this way, dehydration caused by alcohol intake reaches the brain, which is composed of a large amount of water. The unpleasant feeling of a hangover on the day following a night of heavy drinking is mostly from remaining acetaldehyde in the body, but the throbbing headache that lingers is caused by the brain, which has become atrophic from the loss of water in the brain cells. If such heavy drinking is not frequent, the problem of atrophy in the brain may be resolved by drinking enough water. Frequent heavy drinking and the resultant atrophic brain will eventually result in a loss of recovery power, finally reaching a point of diminished brain function. The brains of many alcoholics are atrophic as the result of dehydration from frequent drinking.

Alcohol consumes a large number of enzymes during its breakdown and it is therefore best not to drink. If you must drink, it is recommended that you consume an adequate amount of water both before and after drinking to prevent dehydration.

Smoking causes dehydration

The skin of heavy smokers has a uniquely dark tint and premature sagging. This is due to the aging of skin from chronic dehydration. The fluid in our body consists of intracellular fluid and extracellular fluid. Intracellular fluid is literally fluid inside cells. Extracellular fluid is outside cells, specifically blood plasma and lymph that is fluid between cells. As mentioned earlier, 60-70% of the body is fluid, so about 40% of the body is intracellular fluid and 20% extracellular fluid.

When the body's supply of water is short or when a large amount of fluid is lost, the first loss comes from extracellular fluid such as blood plasma and lymph. As dehydration continues and the amount of extracellular fluid decreases, the body tries to prevent the loss of blood by getting fluid from inside the cells. A decline of intracellular fluid compromises the work of these cells, the production of enzymes and their activities inside the cells. This loss of the volume and activity of enzymes implies the loss of enzyme power to fight oxidation. The reason why dehydration accelerates the aging of cells is because of weakened enzyme power from a shortage of fluid. Thus, in order to stay healthy and youthful, it is important to supply an adequate amount of water and to eliminate the causes of dehydration.

Caffeine in coffee speeds up aging

So far, I have stated that alcohol and smoking cause dehydration. In addition, I would recommend only a very limited intake of caffeine. Caffeine has a strong diuretic property. When you drink a lot of tea or coffee with strong caffeine, you are inviting serious dehydration. Coffee lovers like its stimulating property, but there is a risk involved. Some drink coffee to wake up. Coffee has a property that stimulates the central nervous system. Due to this excessive stimulation to the energy-forming network, you may feel temporarily energized, but excessive intake of coffee can lead to an arrhythmic heartbeat due to the burden to heart muscles.

This excessive production of energy may also lead to the feeling of exhaustion after the burst of energy is gone. The biggest problem of excessive production of energy is the waste of enzymes. If you consider the decline of enzyme power from dehydration and the waste of enzymes by excess production of energy, you will understand why too much caffeine accelerates the aging process. It is wise not to exceed 2 to 3 cups of coffee and tea a day.

Sports drinks during exercise could be risky

As mentioned earlier, thirst is not the first signal to let you know that the water in your body is depleting, but it is a warning to tell you that you are in a dangerous state of dehydration. If you grow plants, you probably know that it is important to water plants regularly before they wither. After watering, they recover, but if you repeat the cycle of watering only after a sign of withering, plants get weaker and eventually die.

The same is true with the human body. There are increasing numbers of people dying from heat strokes in summer, and I think this is an indication that more people are chronically dehydrated. With adequate water you are unlikely to die from dehydration, unless you exert yourself with excessive exercise in the hot sun. In order to live a long life, however, it is more important to prevent problems than to cure them. Similarly, it is far more important to drink an adequate supply of water than to supply it only after a sign of thirst. For sports activity during summer, adequate water before a game will prevent the risk of heat stroke or dehydration. Some amateur golfers avoid drinking water during play, saying that beer tastes best when one is thirsty. This is dangerous. I dare say it is a suicidal act to drink beer which has a diuretic effect when one is dehydrated. If one must drink beer, my suggestion is to drink 500 ml (2-3 cups) of water before drinking beer. Some say they will drink beer first and then water because they both go inside their body anyway. Water consumed after beer is wasted because it is excreted by the diuretic property of beer. That's why it is important to drink water *before* drinking beer.

One reason exercise is good for you is that it stimulates muscles and this facilitates the flow of body fluid., If the blood is thick, however, body fluid cannot flow smoothly. Those people who get tired easily from exercise are most likely deficient in water. With a deficient amount of water, adequate nutrients and oxygen are not supplied efficiently, muscles and cells fail to work fully, and this is why you feel tired. When you are dragging like this, my suggestion is to drink water and lie down for a while. As water is distributed to cells, the body's enzyme power is elevated, thus eliminating the feeling of fatigue. In short, it is important to drink water before exercise, before a meal, before drinking alcohol and *especially* when one feels thirsty.

Some say it is better to drink sports drinks than plain water while playing sports. Certainly it is important to consume not only water but also minerals such as sodium, potassium, magnesium and so forth, because they are lost as sweat. I do not recommend sports drinks, however, because they contain a large amount of sugar in addition to minerals. In a regular soft drink in a bottle of 500ml there are 30-50g sugar. In a sports drink, even more sugar is included for recovery from fatigue. It may be all right if an athlete drinks it during his rigorous exercise to supplement his energy, but for ordinary golfers or joggers, such a drink has too much risk.

It is well known that an excessive intake of soft drinks is the cause of so-called soft drink metabolic syndrome. Sports drinks contain substances to control osmosis for effective absorption. Thus, glucose is absorbed rapidly, elevating blood sugar level. This is why sports drinks have more risk for diabetes than regular soft drinks. The best way to supplement minerals lost by perspiration is to take a pinch of good quality salt with water. A tiny pinch for a glass of water or two is sufficient.

Understand the difference between water and fluid, and between salt and saline

How much water do you drink every day? Remember that water and fluid are two separate entities, so any drink besides plain water doesn't count as drinking water. For instance, drinks such as coffee, tea and juice contain fluid, but they are not water. There must be many people who don't drink water every day. I found many among my patients who had consumed a large amount of coffee, soda, juice and so forth, but not much water. There were those who hardly drank any water. Needless to say, all of those patients were dehydrated, and their skin showed it with the advanced age of its cells. Their health suffered, too. Some had already developed a serious disease such as cancer. I have discussed the risk of sports drinks. Basically, any drink other than water cannot quench the thirst of cells.

Tea and coffee contain a large amount of fluid, and at the same time they contain many natural chemical substances. Coffee contains about 25 varieties of natural chemical substances, and so does tea. In order to get the water necessary for the body from these drinks, it would be necessary for the body to filter out these impurities and to detoxify the body, consuming a large amount of enzymes in the process. The caffeine in coffee and tea is diuretic, and therefore a large portion of the water is lost.

Concentrated juices and other juices produced in factories to stock our grocers' shelves are barely useful for the body because enzymes are destroyed by the processing treatments. Most vitamins are also destroyed. Instead, these juices contain a large number of additives such as sugar, fructose and the like. Excess intake may lead to blood sugar spikes, and that can lead to diabetes or hypoglycemia. Some may think homemade juices, since they have lots of vitamins intact, are safe for quenching thirst, but they also have too much sugar to drink in lieu of water. Keep in mind that some fruits contain diuretic substances such as potassium and citric acid, resulting in a loss of water. Fruits contain good quality enzymes and are good for our health, but it is necessary to supplement them with enough water. In my "7 health methods," I recommend drinking water before eating fruit, not as a dessert after a meal, but as an appetizer before a meal. In other words, drink water, followed by fruits, and then a meal. This is important to prevent dehydration and consumption of enzymes. In order to observe this sequence, I follow this routine to drink water:

Morning	Upon wakening	2–3 cups (500-750ml)
Lunch	1 hour before lunch	2–3 cups (500-750ml)
Dinner	1 hour before dinner	2–3 cups (500-750ml)

In this manner I can consume 1.5-2 liters of water easily. Those who cannot drink a lot can start with 300 ml and gradually increase the volume.

Some say excessive intake of water is not good for health. It is true that excess intake of fluid such as coffee, tea, juice, or soda should be avoided, but I believe you can drink as much water as you want, unless you have kidney-related problems. The best diuretic for your body is water.

As mentioned earlier, an appropriate amount of good quality salt is necessary to maintain the balance of vitamins, minerals, and water in the body.

Just as all fluids are not water, there is an important difference between salt and sodium. Refined salt we use in our diet is 99.5% pure NaCl, or sodium. Natural, unrefined salt contains mostly sodium, but it contains other minerals as well. A good quality natural salt contains potassium, magnesium, iodine and iron in good balance. It is made up of 86.5% sodium and 13.5% of those four other minerals. They are all essential for your body.

Sea salt that is made by evaporating water is an especially good natural salt for your health, and it is rich in minerals.

Distilled water is unnatural

There are quite a number of people both in the U.S. and Japan who only drink distilled water. Those people claim that, since it is free from impurities or minerals, it can purge the body of all excess minerals and impurities. I doubt if this is true. There are electrolytes in body fluid, and the density of these electrolytes is maintained at a constant level. When the volume of fluid declines, or when the density of electrolytes in blood increases, the body increases the volume of fluid by encouraging fluid intake by causing a feeling of thirst. The body also tries to maintain the electrolyte density by increasing the volume of urine or sweat. Besides, distilled water is unnatural. Life on earth was born in the sea and humans are said to trace back to the sea. No living thing can survive in water distilled of all minerals and impurities. How could it be that the water in which fish cannot survive is good water? I believe that the best water for our bodies is fresh water from nature.

Natural spring water springs from the earth after having gone through soil, rock beds, and underground water veins. Famous waters found in many parts of the world are all several hundred years of age, counted from the point when the earth receives water as rain until the point the water flows out from the spring, ready for drinking. Through the course of a long journey underground, natural water has been purified and has absorbed minerals necessary for living beings. No water is natural which is free of minerals. We are a part of nature, and I believe that we should drink natural water; and yet it can be a challenge to find water we can drink safely.

I use a water purifier to create drinking water that is close to ideal water. Tap water contains chlorine to kill bacteria. For drinking water, we need to remove the added chlorine and chemicals, but I feel it is disrespectful to nature to remove the minerals given by nature.

Our bodies are closely tied to the land where we live. The ideal diet will be made up of local foods from one's area, prepared and consumed while they are fresh. For this reason, it is important to keep your land clean. When the land where you live becomes contaminated, produce and water from your land becomes contaminated as well.

There is an expression in Buddhist teachings that says, "The consequence of one's deed is inseparable from the environment in which he lives." We who are suffering from environmental contamination should take this expression seriously. We should keep in mind that truly good waters and foods are those produced from a beautiful, lovingly cared-for environment.

CHAPTER 3

A lifestyle to elevate enzyme power

Why do we feel sleepy when we are full?

After a heavy meal we feel sleepy.

When we get drunk, we feel sleepy.

Also we feel sleepy after exercise, or when exhausted from hard work. Why do we get sleepy?

Sleep is necessary for life. Generally speaking, it is a sign to let the brain rest, but we don't understand exactly how the signal to sleep works. We feel sleepy after a meal because blood rushes to the stomach, and as a result parasympathetic nerves become dominant in the autonomic nervous system, releasing tension in the brain. It is true that eating causes changes in the autonomic nervous system. Considering, however, that we feel sleepy after being intoxicated or after exercise, I suspect that the reason we get sleepy is not necessarily to allow the brain to rest. When I look at this question of why we get sleepy from the point of view of enzyme consumption, the observations are quite interesting.

Eating, drinking alcohol, and exercising all cause the body to consume large numbers of enzymes. When you eat, enzymes are used to digest and absorb nutrition. The more food you consume, the more enzymes are used. I think it is because of the depletion of enzymes that you get sleepy after a hearty meal, while you do not get as sleepy after a moderate meal. When you drink alcohol, a large number of enzymes are consumed breaking down and detoxifying the alcohol. The reason why some drinkers of alcohol fall asleep soon is, in my opinion, that the drinker has only a small number of enzymes to break down alcohol and they get depleted quickly. In physical exercises or in mental exercises enzymes are consumed as well, and that is probably the reason for feeling sleepy after exercise or hard work. In other words, sleep is induced in order to recover depleted body enzymes.

When we fall asleep, the autonomic nervous system is switched from the dominance of sympathetic nerves to the dominance of parasympathetic nerves. Parasympathetic nerves are called the relaxation nerves because they work when one is relaxed. As the body temperature goes down, the energy consumption slows down. Enzymes are used in the activities of all living organisms at all times. They are used when we move our limbs, and they are at work when we use our brains. For example, as you read this type, enzymes are being used. When your brain processes what you have read, enzymes are used, and when you think about what you have read enzymes are also used. Thus, by just closing your eyes, the consumption of enzymes slows down. When you feel tired, if you close your eyes and lie down for a few minutes, you will feel refreshed. I believe this is the result of recovering enzymes. During sleep, when we are lying still with our eyes closed, our respiratory rate decreases and the amount of enzymes spent is very small. I think that the need to conserve and replenish enzymes is a major reason we need regular sleep. We sleep to suppress the consumption of enzymes and at the same time to create more new enzymes.

Sleep is not just for resting the brain

When I say body enzymes get replenished during sleep, you may think that enzymes are produced during the long hours of sleep at night. Enzyme production, however, is not limited to the time while you are asleep. Enzymes are produced at all times, but if you are awake and work for long hours or if you eat a heavy meal or drink too much, in the process consuming enzymes, enzyme production will fall behind consumption. We cannot live without enzymes, and thus it becomes necessary to provide a block of time during which the body can concentrate on enzyme production. I think this is an important role of sleep.

Of course, some enzymes are consumed even during sleep because basic activities to sustain life are continuing. Furthermore, our stomachs and intestines, which are under the control of the parasympathetic nervous system, work more actively during sleep than when we are awake. Why are body enzymes restored while stomachs and intestines are active?

Here is the big secret!

Stomachs and intestines are responsible for our health and youth. The more healthy stomachs and intestines work, the more miracle enzymes are produced. The reason for this has to do with the microorganisms that live in our stomachs and intestines. Your body is inhabited by enormous numbers of microorganisms, most of which are not only beneficial, but are vital for your survival. When I say 'inhabited,' you might think I mean these microorganisms are parasitic, but the relationship the body has with these microorganisms is mutually supportive or symbiotic. Without the work of these microorganisms, you would not be able to meet the requirements of your body's functions.

The number of microorganisms in your body fluctuates daily depending on your environment and your body's needs, but suffice it to say that on any given day there are several hundred trillion living inside you. This is an astronomical number when you consider that the number of cells composing your body is 60 trillion. Enzymes are produced not only by cells, but also by microorganisms to make your life activities possible.

Necessary enzymes are produced through the communications between microorganisms in your body and genes in your cells. Cells in your body get such information as when enzymes should be produced, what type of enzymes you need, and how many enzymes should be produced. They do this by communicating with bacteria in your intestines. I believe there is a high probability that the medium for such communications in your body is fluid. I think this is why a shortage of water in the body leads to a failure to properly produce the necessary enzymes.

The cause of aging in the body is oxidation more than biological age. The most powerful antioxidants are enzymes such as *OD catalase*. In producing this antioxidant enzyme inside of the cells, resident bacteria, especially intestinal bacteria, are involved. With good food and water, the environment inside your intestines improves and cells are hydrated, resulting in smooth triangular communications between enzymes, cells, and microorganisms, including intestinal bacteria. Furthermore, the benefit of such a good internal environment is not limited to increased production of enzymes. The quality of the enzymes produced will also be superior.

Recovery of the body's enzymes during sleep has not been proven at present, but I believe my hypothesis of the existence of miracle enzymes and the recovery of enzymes during sleep will soon be scientifically proven. There are many who will not believe anything unless it is proven scientifically, but as far as our personal life and health is concerned, I believe the voice of the body is the most important authority. Learning to listen to your body is the key to your health. For example, growth hormones have become popular as a rejuvenating hormone and it is known that it is secreted during sleep. Before such a medical discovery was made, people would say that an infant who sleeps a lot grows well. Obviously, people have long known from practical experience about the link between good sleep and growth, even if they didn't know about the secretion of growth hormones during sleep.

When we lose sleep for a few days, our skin looks tired. This is an indication that the purpose of sleep is not limited to resting the brain. The body is telling us that the basic requirements to prevent oxidation and aging of the body are not being met. For youthful skin, you need to provide a good diet, good water, and also adequate sleep to recover and revitalize the body's enzymes.

Napping is the best habit for seniors

For 30 years, I have made it a habit to take a nap after lunch. I used to be too busy to get enough sleep at night. One day, after a busy morning, I felt like I just had to have a nap after lunch. I closed my eyes for 15-20 minutes and awakened to find that I felt surprisingly refreshed.

You may doubt the effect of only 20 minutes of sleep, but I urge you try it. Lie down and completely relax. A short nap after lunch can restore your body.

Now, whenever I feel tired, I lie down and take a nap for 5 to 10 minutes. Despite a busy schedule, I have the energy to organize and give lectures, enjoy music and sports; I attribute this stamina to short, effective naps. As a person ages, it gets more difficult to sleep 7 or 8 hours straight. The reason for this is unknown, but it is common knowledge that older people tend to get up at night to go to the bathroom, or wake up very early in the morning. It could be that the rhythm of the span switching between sympathetic nerves and parasympathetic nerves is getting shorter. If this is the case, it will help to make a habit of taking a nap to maintain health and youthfulness.

The following is an observation based on my own experience. When you make a habit of taking a nap, I think this habit is remembered in your cells as the rhythm of your own personal life. When this personal rhythm has been established, the recovery power from a short nap improves.

Not many Americans (or Japanese) take afternoon naps. There are many in other cultures that regularly take afternoon naps. Siesta time in Spain is well known. Such a custom has taken root in countries where the temperature in the afternoon is high and it was not historically feasible to work. The wisdom of nature is telling us to work in the afternoon only after the body's enzymes are restored. From a medical standpoint, I think an afternoon siesta is an excellent custom. Recently there have been companies in the U.S. that recommend 30-minute naps for their employees, because this has been shown to lead to increased efficiency and fewer accidents in the workplace. This practice of a short nap has been given the name "power nap" by Professor James Marsh, a social psychologist at Cornell University. A power nap should not exceed 30 minutes because, with more sleep time, one will reach a deeper sleep cycle and will feel sluggish after awakening. This sluggishness is an indication that the sleep cycle and the nap are not in sync.

Naps are very effective to restore enzymes, so I advise you to adopt such a habit in your life and increase your power to recover enzymes.

Food that is good for the intestine is good for the brain

A while ago in Japan, fish eyes and fish heads were taken up as foods for the brain because they contain a large amount of DHA (docosahexaenoic acid). It is clear from various studies that DHA in fish oil is beneficial for the body, but it is a mistake to have a meal of fish only. In fact, it is a mistake to eat only one kind of nutritious food. Any good food, if taken out of balance, will bring harm to the body. Fish, when compared to other animal-based foods such as beef, pork, or chicken, is far better because it places a much lighter burden on the stomach and intestines. But consumption beyond 15% of any food in a meal is not advisable. It is important to select foods that are good for your body, but most importantly, to have a balanced meal.

There are many other foods besides fish oil that are good for the brain. Some foods beneficial for the brain are blue fish such as mackerel and sardines, soy products, colorful vegetables, and sea vegetables rich with vitamins and minerals. Among grains, rice and barley are known for their benefits. All of these foods are familiar to the Japanese as they have been in our diet from ancient times. The reason a Japanese meal is considered a healthy meal is because it includes these foods in good balance.

The intestines process nutrition for the brain. Food is absorbed in the intestines, and the nutrients are sent to the entire body. In considering what is good for the brain, this is an important point, because foods which are bad for the intestines can not have a good effect on your brain.

After a short while working as an endoscopy and colonoscopy surgeon, I became very interested in what meals would be beneficial to stomachs and intestines. Over the years, I have come to know that foods good for the stomach and the intestines are good for the entire body. The entire body, needless to say, includes the brain. In other words, what is good for the intestines is good for the brain. By the same token, what is bad for the intestines is bad for the brain. Sugary drinks, alcohol, cigarettes, and overconsumption of animal-based foods, all of which have an adverse affect on the intestines, also have an adverse affect on the brain. Good water, which is important for smooth flow in the stomach and intestines, is most essential for the brain. All the parts in our body are linked. Basically, no food is good for the brain only or good for the stomach and intestines only. Anything which is a hazard to any part of the body has a bad affect on the entire body, although the extent of that affect on each organ may vary.

Caffeine depletes savings in the brain

In Chapter 2, I discussed the mechanisms by which there can be serious damage to the brain from the consumption of alcohol. Caffeine found in coffee and tea can also cause serious damage to the brain. First of all, caffeine has a diuretic property, and thus an excess intake of coffee will lead to dehydration.

The damage from caffeine is not limited to dehydration. Excess consumption of caffeine interferes with the relay of information within your body. This is because caffeine interferes with the work of PDE (phosphodiesterase), which performs the role of a second messenger in the relay of information within the body. PDE is involved in learning and memorizing processes. In other words, caffeine depletes the enzyme that you need to save information in the brain.

Recent experiments have proven that caffeine can damage visual and memory molecules. After this finding, Dr. Batmanghekudj, a pioneer of the water cure, emphasized the danger of coffee intake by Alzheimer's patients and learning-impaired children. The degree of alcohol tolerance varies among people, and as a result there are many people who don't drink at all, but most adults (and many children) drink tea or coffee regularly. The toxic effect of coffee is well known and that is why many people prefer to drink decaf.

You probably know coffee is habit-forming, but it is not well known that there is such a thing as a lethal dose of coffee. Half of the population of adults who weigh 110–130 lb. will die if they consume 10-12 grams of caffeine all at once. A cup of coffee contains about 100 mg, or 1/10th of a gram, of caffeine, so that even the consumption of many cups in a short period of time will not lead to death, but some damage to the body cannot be avoided.

Regular coffee drinkers have become somewhat desensitized to caffeine's stimulation, but, since I hardly drink any coffee, when I have a cup, I can tell clearly that there is a change going on in my body. I experience elevated blood pressure and eye pressure, increased heart rate, and an irregular heartbeat. Other known effects include central nerve stimulation (inhibition of sleep, anxiety, insomnia); weakening of muscles; hyper-secretion of gastric fluid, which speeds up digestion and increases stomach irritation; increase of cholesterol (LDL, TC); increased bowel peristalsis (diarrhea), and other effects.

Alcohol, coffee, and smoking all lead to damage to the homeostatic property of the brain.

As one ages, one often experiences declining memory, such as losing the words one wants to say or a slow reaction time in accessing information one knows. This implies an impaired function for relaying information. This is probably caused by a shortage of brain enzymes.

I recommend moderation in consuming caffeine so that the important PDE in the brain will not be compromised.

Is there a drink to facilitate the work of the brain? Yes, there is: *water*. Good water hydrates the brain, helps the work of enzymes in the brain, and activates them.

Many drink coffee during work. My suggestion is to replace coffee with water. You will think and work better.

Aging is evidence of declining enzyme power

When we detect a sign of aging such as wrinkles, spots, or gray hair, we might concentrate on taking care of these symptoms. We might have a laser treatment to remove the spot, inject hyaluronic acid into wrinkles, or dye our hair. Aging is not limited to these visible changes only, however. And, of course, treating these visible signs of aging will have little effect on actual aging. Aging is going on inside the cells, and this aging of the cells is caused by oxidation. Thus, the best anti-aging method is to elevate the anti-oxidative potency in the body, which means to elevate the potency of the body's enzymes to prevent oxidation. When you see someone who appears healthy and young, you can assume that person has strong enzyme power in his or her body.

I have stated that it is important to increase the body's enzymes to stay healthy, and I have discussed how to prevent the unnecessary consumption of enzymes. Enzyme power is not determined by the number of enzymes alone. The *quality* of these enzymes and their activation levels are also very important factors. There is an expression, "The few and the proud." This applies to enzymes. The consumption of your enzymes will be kept to a minimum if your enzymes have high activation levels. Regrettably, a majority of people are not fully utilizing their own enzyme power. There are many factors preventing the activities of enzymes. For the activities of enzymes, coenzymes such as vitamins and minerals are essential. These coenzymes are carried to our cells by body fluids such as blood. Without a smooth flow of body fluids, the functions of our cells are compromised. In extreme cases we can even die.

How can we improve blood circulation? The most effective means is to drink a sufficient amount of water. With an insufficient water intake, the volume of our body fluid depletes, making the blood thick and compromising its flow. As this dehydration advances, water stored in the cells is used, resulting in the drying up of our cells, which in turn compromises the bodily functions they perform. When sufficient water is supplied, the water retention in blood stays stable and the flow of body fluids will improve. Those people who suffer from poor circulation or swelling tend to reduce water intake, but one should keep in mind that a sufficient amount of water will improve blood circulation and reduce swelling. This is the reason why drinking and smoking are unhealthy: both have an adverse effect on blood circulation. Alcohol leads to dehydration and smoking causes constricted blood vessels.

It is also known that poor circulation in the scalp is involved in developing grey hair. Grey hair is caused by the death of stem cells that produce melanocytes at the roots of the hair in your scalp. The death of these stem cells is the result of poor circulation. According to the research by J. G. Mosley, MD, which was published in the *British Medical Journal* in 1996, smokers were found to be four times more likely to begin greying prematurely compared to nonsmokers.

Another cause for decreasing enzyme power is the lowering of body temperature. The ideal temperature for our enzymes is between 99 and 104 degrees. Our body temperature remains steady by a temperature-regulating center, and when we get sick, the temperature-regulating center issues a fever onset signal.

The body attempts to increase immune power by raising its temperature to induce enzymes to increase their work. A drop of a body's temperature by 1 degree can reduce its immune power by 35%. This is due to the loss of enzyme activities from a decline in the body's temperature. Recent research suggests cancer cells are most active at a body temperature of 95 degrees. There are increasing numbers of people with an average body temperature of 95 degrees, especially among young women. They don't seem to mind this, but at a low body temperature, one is more susceptible to sickness and aging is accelerated.

Most of us take our temperature when we feel sick and feverish. I suggest taking your temperature even when you don't feel sick, so you can take steps to raise it if it is low. Your body's temperature can be improved by adopting a proper diet, getting adequate sleep and rest, practicing proper breathing, and adopting a moderate exercise routine. As we get older our activity level may drop. We may also eat less. When dietary intake decreases, we must pay special attention to the balance of our nutrition. Indulging junk food instead of a healthy meal should by all means be avoided. A balanced plant-based diet is recommended. Those who have difficulties sleeping should adopt naps in their daily cycle to prevent compromised enzyme recovery. The proper way to breathe is abdominal breathing through one's nose. When you breathe deeply, you will feel as if the body temperature is rising, and this is because the greater amount of oxygen increases metabolism. Deep breathing through the mouth will result in an increased amount of evaporation of fluids from the body and should be avoided. As for exercise, a light routine is recommended rather than a rigorous one in order to avoid excessive consumption of enzymes. A daily walk may be a good idea.

Another advantage if you want to activate enzymes is happiness. Don't worry, be happy! Enzymes are activated when a person feels love and appreciation. I will discuss this point in the next chapter, but in short, one should make an effort to have a positive frame of mind. It is true that aging is the process of the oxidation of cells, but taking care of your body alone will not bring true health or youthfulness unless you feel happy. Since aging is actually the deterioration of enzymes' power to resist oxidation, the best anti-aging method is to elevate the enzyme power from inside by caring for your body and mind and spirit.

Let's lead a life for healthy soil

The health of each cell of our bodies is impacted by what goes on in our entire body. Our health is similarly impacted by the soil on which we live. The contamination of air, water and soil will lead to the contamination of our bodies. We attempt to protect ourselves from the harmful effects of environmental contamination by buying devices to filter the air and purify the water, but these solutions are like the injection of hyaluronic acid to improve wrinkles. They do not get to the root of the problem. It is my belief that we must start cleaning our natural environment in order to attain real health.

In cleaning up our environment, we might start with cleaning up the soil. Good soil is necessary for healthy plants and healthy food. Contamination of the soil implies contamination of our food. It also implies contamination of our drinking water, even when that water comes from a fresh spring. It is the soil which purifies the rain, adding necessary minerals. In other words, the earth is a natural water purifier. Obviously, contaminated soil will contaminate the water.

In a broad sense, it is also the soil that cleans the air. Trees which clean the air are nourished by the earth, and rain water washes away the dirt in the air, before it in turn gets purified in its journey through the earth. Everything is purified through the intermediation of the earth. All living organisms are part of the environmental system through the intermediary of the earth. Animals eat plants grown on the earth; wastes from animals return to the earth, are broken down by the earth, and become fertilizer for plants.

The earth is involved in the cycling of living organisms, water, and air. Such cycles are made possible by soil bacteria. There are many microorganisms in the soil, and the cycling system of the earth is made possible by their work. It is not an overstatement to say that the earth is a planet of microorganisms. The area where they live stretches from the height of 10,000 meters above ground to the depth of several thousand meters in the soil on land or 10,000 meters in the ocean.

Microorganisms live in an environment that is too harsh for the survival of animals or plants, and they also live inside all animals and plants in the form of parasites or symbiotic microbes.

Truly, we exist in a sea of microorganisms, and microorganisms have a strong impact on our health. In fact, when the balance in our intestinal bacteria is compromised, we suffer from diarrhea or constipation. In the worst case, a change in the balance of microorganisms in our bodies can lead to various types of diseases. The same is true with the earth. If the balance of microorganisms gets out of sync, the recycling system of the earth is impacted. An environmental contamination is a contamination of vital microorganisms in the soil.

With the advancement of civilization, there has been a great advance in medical science. At the same time, there are increasing numbers of people suffering from intractable diseases or unusual diseases. In 1973 there were about 10,000 people suffering from what were called intractable or rare diseases. The same investigation in 2003 found over 500,000 people suffering from such diseases, an astounding increase of 500 percent.

There are many possible environmental causes for such an increase. I am afraid that toxic environmental contamination, including the contamination of microorganisms, is responsible for this sudden increase. It is we who are responsible for upsetting the balance of microorganisms on the earth. We should rethink the use of pesticides and chemical fertilizers in agriculture, the release of polluted water containing chemicals into the ocean and the burying of untreated waste underground so that contaminants leach into the underground streams that feed our drinking water supply.

We have learned a lot from nature, but there are many things in nature we have not come to understand. It is arrogant to think that the science we know can solve all our problems. We should have more respect for the natural order of things and have more appreciation and consideration for microorganisms.

Coexistence with microorganisms improves our enzyme power

Microorganisms have a very short life cycle and are sensitive to environmental changes or external stimulations. For example, MRSA (methicillin resistant Staphylococcus aureus) is a fungus with properties resistant to antibiotics that evolved from staphyloccus aureus after repeated exposures to antibiotics. In other words, it is a monster fungus accidentally created by humans when we upset the natural balance of microorganisms with antibiotics. If, in order to achieve a short term gain, we continue to use pesticides, fertilizers, and antibiotics which are hazardous to the environment, toxic to the soil, and disruptive to microorganisms, then the soil and the mircroorganisms we live with will change properties to adapt to this disruption. The impact of such evolved bacteria on the human body is still unknown, but there is a danger that a monstrous fungus worse than MRSA could be created. The reason why there are increasing numbers of intractable or strange diseases may be partially attributable to changes in fungi. In order to minimize these dangers, it is necessary for us to devise ways to process contaminated substances or break down toxins in a manner in harmony with natural laws.

Consider the way nature breaks down toxins. The process is similar to the way the body breaks down toxins. In nature, enzymes break toxins into substances that are no longer toxic. In soil, various bacteria perform this function. Soil detoxification is carried out in most cases not by a single microorganism but by the power generated by a coalition of microorganisms.

Researchers have recently recognized the potential for using a coalition of microorganisms to create new "green" products that are harmless to the human body and to the environment. These products are created by cultivating hundreds of useful bacteria. Harnessing the power of microorganisms creates products with a range of applications. They can be used to improve soil as well as to break down and clean up various contaminants. At present, waste-water from homes and factories passes through sewage lines and is processed with microorganisms at sewage-treatment plants. After adding chlorine for disinfection, the water is returned to nature. If the waste-water contains a large amount of chemicals such as surfactant, the waste water itself can kill the microorganisms which are used for treating the water which compromises the effectiveness of the water treatment. The new products made by using complex microorganisms could more effectively perform detoxification and purification at the processing plant.

We tend to value things based on their usefulness to us. For example, we classify intestinal bacteria as good bacteria and bad bacteria, and then we try to get rid of the "bad guys." In reality, however, bad bacteria are also indispensable for the proper function of the body. An excess number of bad bacteria is undesirable, but their existence is necessary to maintain a proper balance in our intestines. In the same way, insects we deem useless are called pests and inedible plants are called weeds. This is a self-centered way of thinking, and this mindset makes it difficult to see the advantages of being in harmony with nature and co-existing with microorganisms.

Many microorganisms are involved in the maintenance of human health. Fungi, for example, have taken residence in our bodies. They are brought into our bodies with the foods we eat or the air we breathe. Various types of fungi co-exist inside us, and we have hardly begun to identify which fungus produces which enzyme that contributes to our health. Developed societies are known for their meticulous cleanliness. This is a good quality, but, paradoxically, sterilizing everything is damaging our health. Excessive sterilization will cause the death of fungi that our bodies need. It is important to create an environment where we utilize the power of microorganisms and let the microorganisms in the body exert their power.

Why pianists live long lives

There is a saying that goes, "Few physicians live well." When I look around, there are quite a number of physicians who fall ill at an early age or worry too much about their retirement, and they age suddenly. It could be said that the work of physicians is hard, both physically and mentally, and that their consumption of their enzymes may therefore be greater than with other people.

There are some professions where people enjoy an especially long, active career and who also have long lives. The most notable is that of musicians. The world famous conductors, pianists, and violinists lead busy lives, performing all over the planet, and yet many stay youthful despite advancing age.

Why are there many musicians who live a long life? Some say, "It is because they use their fingers." It is true that the use of fingers stimulates the brain, activating brain enzymes. I doubt if that is the only reason for the long, healthy life of musicians. If the use of fingers is the cause, typists, computer programmers and other professionals using their fingers should live long as well. Among medical physicians, surgeons are required to have delicate finger technique but they do not as a rule live as long.

Why do musicians live longer? My theory is that the mind is involved in music. Musicians use their fingers while enjoying the vibrating sound of their favorite music, and because of this joy, enzyme activation is multiplied many times. As a hobby, I play the flute and other instruments and know that playing music is a great way to create a happy state and to relieve stress. I get much enjoyment from playing music, and when I play well after repeated practices, I feel flooded with happiness. I am busy with my professional work, and I cannot spare time until it is quite late at night. I feel tired and sleepy, but when I start playing the flute, I become relaxed and am filled with happiness. When I go to bed after an hour's practice, I can get up the following morning feeling refreshed, probably from the elevated level of enzyme power.

When I feel tired and go straight to bed, skipping the practice, I don't feel as refreshed when I wake up the next morning.

In modern medicine, people tend to regard body and mind as separate entities, but they cannot be approached separately. No matter how beneficial a practice you employ for your body may be, you cannot realize full enzyme power if your mindset is negative. It is important to live your life from your heart. This does not just apply to the practice of music. The same is true with meals and exercises. You should enjoy a meal that is good for your body and enjoy exercise that moves and strengthens your body. When you enjoy and appreciate a meal, the microorganisms and cells in your body appreciate the meal as well, and this elevates your enzyme power. If you exercise with joy, the effect on your body will be multiplied. In short, the best way to elevate enzyme power is to engage with joy activities that are good for your health.

CHAPTER 4

Young mind, young body

Visit by a mafia boss on the second day of my practice

On the second day after I opened my clinic in New York back in February, 1972, I received a patient, the 22nd patient in my practice. This man was from Philadelphia and was dressed all in black. He was accompanied by his wife and 10 very large, muscular men who were also clad in black. I felt as if I were in a scene from "The Godfather."

The presence of 10 men clad in black in my small waiting room was too much, so I asked them to wait outside. I received the man and his wife in my examination room. When I asked the man, "Is anything wrong?," he did not hesitate to reply, "While I was serving time in the penitentiary, I had numerous bouts of rectal bleeding. The bleeding was heavy and each time I had to receive a transfusion of 5 to 6 units of blood." One unit contains 500 milliliters of blood, and thus he had received 2.5 to 3 liters of blood each time he had this episode.

This is a considerable amount of blood.

He continued, "I was examined in a university hospital and was told I had severe diverticulitis in my intestines, but they could not tell which diverticulum was causing bleeding and they said I had to have my entire intestine removed. But I don't feel convinced this is necessary. Then I heard about you. I understand you can look inside an intestine without abdominal surgery. Can you do this and find out where I am bleeding?"

In July, 1968 I had developed the first successful technique for removing polyps without an abdominal incision, using a snare wire connected to a colonoscope. Since then I have taught many physicians who wanted to learn the technique. Such a technique demands a very high degree of skill. Intestines with diverticulitis are hard and narrow, and often there are adhesions, making it more difficult to examine the entire intestine. There is a major risk of perforation. In early 1972, I was still the only surgeon who had mastered such a technique in the entire country, and that was why this Mafia boss had come from Philadelphia to see me.

Some in my office suggested that I should decline his request with some excuse, because he was a mafioso, and things could become complicated. I had made up my mind when I became a physician to treat all patients, and so I accepted his request, although I admit I was a little scared. A few days later, I examined inside his intestine using the colonoscope and was shocked. He had told me he had diverticulitis, but the condition of his intestine was far worse than I expected. There were numerous diverticula scattered about in the sigmoid, descending colon, ascending colon, transverse colon, and even in the cecum. In such a condition, a majority of the colon must be taken out unless the bleeding spots are identified and removed. As I was very carefully examining him, I found a trace of bleeding at a location about one meter from the anus. I advised him that I identified the location of bleeding and recommended an open abdominal surgery and a removal of about 30cm of the right side colon where it was bleeding. I further advised him that physical damage could not be avoided, but when compared with the option of having the entire colon taken out, a partial removal would be a much better option. He did not decide right away, and told me he would return on the following day.

Three wishes gone awry

I was 36 years old. I was recognized in the medical field for my skill in polypectomy using a colonoscope, but I had just started my own practice, and the patient was a Mafia boss well known in the U.S. I thought the surgery should be performed by a more experienced physician in the field, and I thus prepared for the meeting with the patient on the following day with such a recommendation.

At the meeting the Mafia boss stated, "My wife and I would like you to operate." I was shocked, and I blurted out, "In New York, there are many distinguished surgeons who are known for their skills with this operation. You should be asking those doctors." Their reply was, "We have checked on you, Dr. Shinya. We have learned that you used to operate as a resident physician for your supervising physician and that you have a reputation as a doctor with skillful hands." Thus, shortly after I opened my first practice, I was to operate on this Mafia don. He was 65 years old and the operation would not be an easy one. Fortunately, however, the operation was successful and he made a smooth recovery.

Despite my young age he trusted me and followed my instructions diligently in the post-operation care. We came to talk about many things whenever I examined him, and soon after he got out of the hospital, he started inviting me for dinner at his home. He turned out to be a charming dinner host, with gentlemanly behavior and a good sense of humor. We talked about my future and my dream to make a contribution to health and medicine. He told me he would support me.

About a year later, while we were dining, he said, "You saved my life. I have recovered completely. I have decided to transfer all my work to my son and start my second life quietly with my wife. I have also decided to take the witness stand, which the police have been asking me to do for some time, to make a settlement with my past. I owe it to you."

I was very pleased. A patient I took care of now cared for his body and wanted to make similar improvements in all aspects of his life. He continued, "I would like to give you a gift as a token of my appreciation. If you had three wishes what would your wishes be?" We were having dinner, and I decided to play along for fun.

I said, "A 10-carat diamond; 100 acres of land in Florida, and I cannot think of a third one. I'll come up with something by the time we meet next," and we laughed.

Regrettably the next meeting never took place. Shortly after this dinner conversation, I read in the newspaper that he had been shot in front of his house in Philadelphia and was dead. A gift of a diamond and 100 acres of land was a humorous dinner fantasy, but what this patient actually gave me was much more precious. The trust he had in me at the start of my career gave me the courage I needed to develop and practice my skills. Many people who heard about me from him visited my clinic. It is very regrettable that he died soon after he recovered his health and his life, but I came to believe that he found peace at the end.

Some people shut their minds, some open their minds

A woman visited my clinic several years ago. She was 42 years of age and told me she was a medical doctor specializing in internal medicine and nutritional science. She was dressed well, but looked older than her age. She held herself aloof, without any hint of a smile. Diagnosed as having inoperable breast cancer, she came to see me for an examination of her colon and for prescriptions for supplements I recommended.

Often women diagnosed with breast cancer and men diagnosed with prostate cancers have poor intestinal features. In some instances they also have developed colon cancers in addition to their other cancer. This patient knew that I had been advocating early colon examinations. When I examined her colon, I found it was hard, narrow, and impacted with dry mucous membranes in dark color. Although rigid with spasms and in a poor state, her colon had no perceivable cancer yet. Still, I was concerned that her condition would worsen if nothing was done.

From my experience, this kind of colon is the result of a diet with a large consumption of dairy food with low fat content, such as cottage cheese. I suspected that her diet would fall under this category and asked her about her diet, a question I always ask my patients. Suddenly she became angry. "I am not an ordinary patient. I don't have to tell you my dietary habits. I might say I have studied nutrition much more than you have."

Her burst of her anger caught me by surprise. I apologized, saying, "I am sorry, but I make it a practice to take a dietary history of all my patients. It helps me understand the correlation between diet and the condition of the intestines. I asked her again if she would contribute to this study." She would not reply. She purchased the supplements I prescribed and left without a smile. She did not return to my clinic. Probably she blamed herself for falling ill in spite of her physician's training. I believe she died not too long after. Had she understood the need for changing her diet and lifestyle, perhaps her approach to fighting cancer might have been quite different. It is regrettable, but it is impossible to cure a person with a closed mind, even if that person is a medical doctor.

In order to conquer a disease, it is absolutely necessary to keep an open mind. No one else can do this for us. It is up to us to be open-minded and willing to change. My approach was the same both with the Mafia boss who opened his mind and the female physician who shut her mind off. The difference was in their willingness to see only what they already believed.

Diagnostic process with an interview enhances recovery and immunity

I receive many new patients referred by other physicians and other patients of mine. They don't feel quite well and want to find out if anything is wrong. When I detect a serious problem such as cancer, I always ask, "What do you think the cause of your problem is?" You may think it is odd for a physician to ask a patient about the cause of his disease. This is, however, a very important question for a patient to answer for himself when dealing with his illness. Those who suspect their disease is coming from excessive drinking or smoking, irregular life patterns, or exhaustion from hard work are relatively frank and talk about these things.

"I used to drink every day."

"I cannot quit smoking."

"The work load for the past few years has been heavy. I must have over-exhausted myself with work."

Those who feel that their physical problems are caused by their mental or emotional problems will usually not speak out. They are hesitant to talk to a third party, such as myself, about these very private matters. I try to help them, saying, "You can talk about anything. Once you unload what is on your mind, you will feel better." I offer to make time to listen to their problems. "Please try to talk about it," I encourage them. Mutual trust is important for the relationship between a medical doctor and a patient, and in order to gain such trust, both must keep an open mind.

I try to talk with my patients about lots of subjects. Many of my patients have been coming to my clinic for routine checkups regularly for many years. I don't want to end an examination by simply saying, "I did not find any polyps or cancer so please come again in 2 years." It is my belief that a physician's job is not limited to a physical examination. Physical examination is only 50% and the remaining 50% is paying attention to the state of mind of each patient through conversation. This is because I know that the mind has a great affect on the body.

I always explain the results of my examinations. Merely stating that there are no polyps or that there is cancer will not reach the patient's mind. I explain the condition of his colon which I just examined, if it is better or worse compared with the result of the previous examination, and, if appropriate, ask about what he has done to improve his diet and his health. Then I praise him for the efforts he has made.

If his condition is worse, I ask what may have caused the deterioration. I might say, "When I examined your colon today, it was a little dry. Your face also looks a little dry. How much water do you drink in a day? Isn't your blood pressure a little higher recently? When you don't have enough water, your blood pressure goes up. You should drink about this much water," and I show him what he should do. When I don't see any physical cause for a patient's complaints, I ask if there has been any change in his life. If he is a golf lover, I will talk about the course I recently played so that he will feel comfortable enough to talk about himself. With such an approach, even those people who are shy or very private often begin to open up after a few visits and start talking and smiling. A patient with an open mind is easier for me to treat, and the effect of the treatment will be seen sooner. I believe that the mind that feels free to trust and to share with others will activate enzymes, and as the result that person's immune power will be elevated.

Doctors should never tell patients how long they have to live

No matter how serious the finding from an examination is, I never lie to my patients. Sometimes family members ask me not to tell the patient about the problem. In such an instance, I try to convince the family members of the importance of sharing the truth. It may sound strange, but patients with diseases such as cancer who accept the reality, including the possibility of death, are often cured. It is important to accept one's condition and, at the same time, not to despair about it. The reason I ask my patients about the cause of her condition is to help her understand and accept her disease.

After hearing my diagnosis, some ask how much time they have left. I always answer with the truth: "I don't know." You must have watched a scene on television where a doctor tells a patient that he has three months left to live, but I believe it is a mistake for a doctor to make such a statement. My answer is, "Your life is God-given. You are asking me when God will call you and that is not something I can know."

I tell the truth to a patient because I believe that can help him lead a better life. This is different from saying he does not have much time left, because then a patient will accept his death rather than his life. There is a very big difference. The deeper the trust between a patient and his doctor, the more the patient will be affected by what his doctor says. When a doctor's prediction comes true for a patient, people may be impressed with the accurate prediction of the doctor, but it may well be the result of auto-suggestion on the part of the patient, after he has heard the doctor's words.

All people will die at some point. The reason one is ill may be the result of lifestyle choices that did not properly take care of the body, but when one has fallen ill, it is more important to accept the reality of the situation and make the rest of one's life more fulfilling than to regret past behavior and decisions. Mr. B., the Mafia boss I mentioned earlier, faced his disease and recovered his health but lost his life to a gunshot wound. And yet, he had taken care of his body and decided on a new course for his life. I believe that was truly meaningful and redemptive for him.

The mind has boundless power

In general, physical strength refers to endurance or stamina. I believe, however, that the source of physical strength is enzyme power. When your enzyme power diminishes, your physical strength diminishes, and when your enzyme power recovers, your physical strength recovers. I cannot help but think there is "heart-and-mind power" comparable to physical power, and that both are vital for life.

Heart-and-mind power is the fundamental power of being human. Sometimes it is called heart, or will; it involves a force much deeper than intellect alone. We speak of "winning hearts and minds" to a cause. My years of experience have taught me that my mind/will/heart has boundless power. I became a medical doctor because I wanted to be a medical doctor in my mind and heart. I have written books because, in my mind and heart, I wanted to relay important things to as many people as possible.

In Chapter 1, I stated that those who look youthful are those who want to stay youthful. This is an example of heart-and-mind power. Heart-and-mind power can be generated regardless of one's physical condition. If you have a clear mindset and decide on an objective, you can exert your heart-and-mind power instantly. Again, what I mean by heart-and-mind power is different from mental power or intellect. You can cultivate physical strength or intellect by yourself. You can develop physical power through diligent exercises. You can elevate your mental power through meditation, spiritual concentration, or by pursuing your goal through study and work.

Heart-and-mind power, however, cannot be achieved by yourself. Heart-and-mind power is the power of love, which will grow by opening your mind and giving love to people around you.

When moved by love, your wish to look young is not selfish. A person living on a deserted island would not care about looks. It is important for me to stay youthful in my appearance in order to gain trust as a medical doctor who wants to teach others about preventive medicine. Actresses and heads of state want to look youthful because they want to appear attractive and full of life force before their audiences.

Heart-and-mind power is generated only by a desire to be of help to others, to connect with others heart-to-heart. "Grandma, stay healthy," from a grandchild; a father's "I believe in you"; an "I love you" from a significant other—I think everyone has had an experience when someone showed them love and elevated their heart-and-mind power, washing away fatigue and fear. A girl in love starts glowing visibly when she is loved in return. I believe this is due to heart-and-mind power. An old man marries a young woman and gets rejuvenated because he has a strong desire to be youthful for his wife.

There are cases in which a man miraculously recovers from a hopeless physical state. In such an instance, there is always love from someone around him as well as his own love for those around him that elevates his heart-and-mind power. Probably, enzymes are energized by the power of love, and the healing and recuperative powers in his body are exerted to the maximum degree. Such healing power and recuperative forces are far more powerful than physical intervention or medicines. How many people can you count to whom you can give your love? The more you love, the stronger the heart-and-mind power generated. If you have very few to love or if you have none, it means that you have not opened your heart and mind to people around you.

I suggest you open your heart and mind and smile and talk to others with love.

Retirees with a positive outlook become rejuvenated

In my 70s, I spend time in the kitchen when I entertain my friends or help my family. The first time I worked in a kitchen was the year when I entered elementary school. When I watched my mother, who had a weak constitution, getting up early and preparing lunch boxes for her children, I decided to help her and to cook rice in the morning.

These days cooking rice is easy, if you have a rice cooker. You merely need to wash rice, put it in a rice cooker, add water according to the directions, and turn on the cooker switch. In those days, however, there was no rice cooker and there was not even a gas stove. I had to gather firewood and cook in a furnace. Of course, it was necessary to attend to it in order to adjust the heat. It was a new task for a child in the first grade of elementary school, and I made a mess in the beginning. My mother never got angry when I made a mistake, and she taught me how to get rid of the burnt smell by using charcoal. When there was not enough water I learned to add a small cup of rice wine to make it fluffy.

I think I owe it to my mother that I became interested in food and that I enjoy cooking and am aware of the importance of meals. I continued cooking rice in the morning until I reached the fifth grade. My mother was very pleased and I felt happy that my attempt to help was lovingly appreciated. My effort to help my mother was returned to me as my own happiness.

When you give love to people around you, it has a therapeutic effect not only for the people you love, but also for yourself.

My mother used to say to me, "Become a fine doctor like Dr. Hideyo Noguchi when you grow up." My desire to live up to my mother's expectations is still a strong motivation for my work of bringing health to as many people as I possibly can. They say it is important to set a goal in order to enrich one's life, and I agree. From my childhood my goal was to become a good medical doctor who could cure disease. I achieved my goal of becoming a medical doctor, and I learn more every day about how to help the body stay well and how to cure its disease. My deep motivation is based on love and on meeting my mother's expectations.

There are many types of motivation. For some people, it is money, status, responsibility, or even anger. A far stronger motivation, however, would be based on eternal love. For example, a President may age rapidly after his retirement because he has achieved his goal and lost his motivation. His drive to become President and his drive to play a strong role in this position after he is elected are his motivations and they are what gives purpose to his life. Once his term is over and he has fulfilled his goal, his drive is gone.

Many wage earners age suddenly after retirement for the same reason. If the motivation to become President or pursue a career was the love of making the lives of many people better, then the President or any retired person would remain active serving others within the scope of his ability. A good example of this is Jimmy Carter, who received a Nobel Peace prize for his work in the two decades *after* he was retired as President. When we retire, we should not take it negatively, even if we are voted out of office, as Jimmy Carter was. We should meet retirement with a positive outlook and think that the time has come to start a new life for family, for oneself and for others. In this way, you will not age suddenly but could instead be rejuvenated.

For those in love, sex is the best rejuvenation secret

The Japanese, like some Americans, tend to regard sex as taboo, but I think it is important to enjoy sex because it is an act of ultimate compassion. I think the expression "make love" is beautiful because it shows the importance of the role of sex in a happy life.

I find it baffling that so many people are embarrassed about the act of sex. The declining sexual relationship between married couples after only a few years together is taken as a social issue in Japan these days. I think that negative attitudes toward sex may have something to do with such a trend.

One of the values of a human is to be happy, and sex is very important in bringing us personal happiness. The value of sex between two people is not just procreation. Sex is an act of ultimate consideration toward the partner. Age is not an issue. According to a survey by the *Harvard Health Letter,* the statistics of those who had sex on a regular basis were as follows: 81% among women in their 60's, 65% in their 70's; 91% for men in their 60's and 79% in their 70's. More importantly, over 90% of those active sexually remained in good health.

Sex and health are interrelated. That is easy to understand when you know that sex regulates hormonal balance and improves blood flow. Naura Hayden, a writer and nutritionist, wrote in her book that a fulfilling sex life will slow aging and maintain youthfulness for women. I am a little disappointed that she does not mention the same thing for men. I suspect the consumption of enzymes from ejaculation may be the answer. An ancient Chinese book on sex reads, "In intercourse, do not ejaculate." Young people need not pay any attention to this, but for men with advancing age, this is a good teaching. If a man refrains from frequent ejaculations, sex is also a good means for rejuvenation. I am by no means recommending sexual activities for the sake of gaining youthfulness. I just want to emphasize that sex with love is an effective means for a couple to show their love, open their hearts and minds, and enrich their lives.

Diagnosis for "menopausal syndrome" is not reliable

Women at menopausal age often suffer from dizziness, palpitations, cold sweats, fluctuating blood pressure, buzzing in the ear, stomach aches, diarrhea, and mild fever. When they go to a doctor about these symptoms, they are diagnosed for menopausal syndrome. It is generally believed that menopausal syndrome is caused by the fluctuation in the secretion of estrogen during a menopausal period. It is true that the hormonal balance may become erratic during a menopausal period and hot flashes ensue, but I think there are other factors involved. First of all, a diagnosis of "menopausal syndrome" for any symptom is too cursory. I think there are other causes for these symptoms. Some women suffer from them while others are not affected. Among those with the syndrome, the extent of such discomfort varies. If imbalance in estrogen were the only cause, it would be unlikely that there would be such a variation of symptoms.

During a menopausal period, changes are not limited to menstruation; there are various changes taking place in a woman's body. For example, the production of SOD, a well known antacid, starts declining. With this change, the damage from an irregular lifestyle will surface as stomach aches and diarrhea.

Many of the diseases now referred to as "lifestyle diseases" used to be labeled "adult diseases" because they are mostly found among adults. With the increasing onset of such symptoms among young people, further studies were conducted, and it was determined that these symptoms are caused by certain lifestyle choices; the name was thus changed from "adult-onset" to "lifestyle."

I think the same could be true of menopausal syndrome. I think there is a likelihood that symptoms surface as the result of an unhealthy lifestyle and are not caused by menopause. In fact, the menopausal syndrome has recently been found among men. Also, there are instances in which young women develop the same syndrome from sudden dietary changes. Thus, I don't buy the diagnosis for "menopausal syndrome." It is not the age of the woman that is causing the problem, but the quality of her lifestyle—factors such as diet, water intake, and elimination of waste among other things. I urge those suffering from menopausal syndrome and those who are approaching menopause to improve their quality of life by practicing my health method. With a sufficient amount of miracle enzymes and good hydration, the process of hormonal changes will be smooth. I am certain that those who are truly healthy will not experience menopausal syndrome.

Characters prone to disease and characters not prone to disease

I try to spend a considerable time talking with my patients. In most cases I take their dietary information myself. Sometimes, my nurses tell me that they should get this information because many patients are waiting for an examination while I'm spending too much time chatting and telling jokes. I will not give up this informal time with my patients, however, because I am not merely collecting data. All the information I am getting in these face-to-face meetings is necessary for a true diagnosis. Through conversation, I learn a patient's character and constitution. For example, we administer premedication to a patient before a colonoscopy to reduce the physical and mental burden on the patient. This is different from anesthesia, but it will make the body relax, inducing sleep.

After an examination is over, I always ask the patient how the medication was. Some say, "It was very pleasant. It felt so good I am waiting to come back for another one." Such a person needs my attention because, if he feels pleasure from premedication, he could be susceptible to dependence on alcohol or drugs. For those people, we use lesser amounts of the medication on his next examination and pay special attention to his prescriptions. Those prone to such reactions to drugs are more easily addicted, and it is important to keep this in mind when inquiring about dietary habits. If I advise the patient not to take any alcohol or to quit drinking, he may lie about the volume of his alcohol consumption.

People know that alcohol is not good for their health, and they thus change their answers depending on the way questions are asked or how I react to their answers. It is very important to know a patient's character and temperament in order to get accurate data. In the course of these interviews with people of different dispositions, I have come to know that there is a connection between one's disposition and one's health. The impression I get, based on my experience, is that people with a cheerful and positive disposition rarely suffer from serious diseases, while those with a negative disposition or those who focus on details are more likely to suffer from diseases.

The following data by Dr. Hans Eysenck is an interesting comment on personality and disease profile:

Type A (Aggressive)

They are competitive, pressed for time and unable to relax. In human relations, they exhibit assertiveness and are competitive. They tend to make deliberate efforts, resulting in increased stress and are thus prone to heart diseases, high blood pressure and strokes.

Type B (Balanced)

They are characterized for their ability to be neutral. They don't feel pressed by time and are not concerned with desire and ambition. They don't want to work all day, every day. In short, they are laid-back types.

Type C (Cancer)

They suppress their emotion and are patient. They don't show their grief or uncertainty, but internalize them. This type is often found among those nice people who prioritize harmony with people around them. When one suppresses his feelings, his stress level goes up and he is prone to depression. As a result, his immune power deteriorates, leading to a probability of the onset of cancer.

It is never too late

Sometimes, you hear, "He used to take such good care of his health. How could he have come down with such a disease?"

We are talking about a person who cares very much about his health; someone who regularly exercises, eats organic vegetables, uses a water purifier, and takes various types of supplements to avoid illness, and yet this fervent pursuer of health has developed cancer. Some of my patients are so serious in their efforts at health that I have to advise them not to be paranoid. These people become ill, not from their lifestyle or negligence in their diets, but because of their very self-centered focus on perfecting themselves. People who are anxious perfectionists about health cannot attain health, no matter how diligently they tend to their bodies, because negative emotions such as worry, uncertainty, sorrow, envy, or anger deplete enzyme power.

In order to enjoy health, one needs to feel happy. It is important to care for your body, but it is more important to care for your spirit. I don't do anything I don't like, either in my work or in my private life.

Some may say, "You can get away with that because you are a doctor, but I am a salaried employee, and often I have to do things I don't like."

Is it really true that most people have to do things they don't want to do?

If, in your job, you produce the good results expected of you, you will be appreciated and will enjoy your work. If you are not appreciated or continually forced to do things you do not like, then a change of jobs might be the answer. I was not an independent practitioner all my life. I was an intern and an associate in lower-level work in university hospitals, but I did not do what I did not like. I worked really hard, although nobody told me to, because I was working for my own satisfaction and happiness.

When I was 18 years old and preparing for admittance to a medical university, I heard a talk by a grand champion of Sumo wrestling. He said, "In order to become a champion, you must have skill with both your right hand and your left hand." I had already made up my mind to be a physician and a surgeon. I took what he said to heart and told myself, "I must be able to use surgical scissors and knives with either hand." I embarked on a daily practice learning to use both my hands equally until I was able to cut a piece of paper along a line with one hand and sew a piece of fabric with another. Because of this practice I mastered a technique using both hands that would serve me well in the operating room. My colleagues used to call me "Miracle Hands" when I was a resident physician in an American hospital.

I go to bed listening to a tape of English words. I do this partly so as not to forget those difficult words that we seldom use, but at the same time I enjoy the beautiful sound of the tape. I play the flute, I play golf, I read medical reports and spend time on research work every day, because all of these things make me happy.

I don't recommend any health maintenance method or anti-aging method if you hate it and do it only as a task to reach an objective. Your healthy practice or anti-aging practice exists as a means to enrich your life and add joy to the years you share with someone you love. The damage to a body from meat consumption is different depending on the state of your mind. There is a big difference between eating a steak with a sense of guilt thinking, "This is not good for my stomach and intestines," as opposed to eating it thinking, "This is delicious and I am so happy."

The power of hearts and minds based on love is absolute. If you awaken your heart-and-mind power and continue doing things beneficial for your body, a favorable change will follow, even if you are sick now and there are various signs of aging and decline. It is true, however, that it is not easy to maintain your joy at its full potential all the time. A mere comment or a trifling incident can sometimes depress your feelings. An occasional poor mood is normal and nothing to worry about. Try to remember the joy when you feel happy, and when you feel down tell yourself it is all right because it will be better tomorrow. This way you direct your mind towards happiness.

It is not too late yet. I would like you to remember that your enzyme power is at the highest level when you love, appreciate, feel pleased and grateful, and make an effort to choose happiness and joy. Each of us can create a happy life by caring for the people who are in our life. You can regain a young, flexible mind and a fresh, vigorous, active body.

Preface from *The Enzyme Factor*

I came of age in Japan just after the war, when American technologies and customs were transforming my native land. I wanted to study medicine in America. I took a medical degree in Japan and then, in 1963, moved to the United States with my young bride to start the surgical residency program at the Beth Israel Medical Center in New York.

Coming to the U.S. from a foreign country, I understood that I had to try hard and be really good to be respected as a surgeon in America. Growing up, I had studied martial arts and, because of that training, I learned to use each hand equally well. Being ambidextrous enabled me to perform surgery with unusual efficiency.

During my residency, I assisted Dr. Leon Ginsburg, one of the discoverers (with Drs. Burrill Bernard Crohn and Gordon Oppenheimer) of Crohn's disease. One day the chief resident and the senior resident who usually assisted Dr. Ginsburg couldn't assist in the operating room, so Dr. Ginsburg's nurse, who had seen me work, recommended me. Being ambidextrous, I finished very quickly. At first Dr. Ginsburg couldn't believe it was done correctly in such a short operation and he was angry, but when he saw how well the patient healed without the excessive bleeding and swelling that follows a lengthy surgery, he was impressed. I started working with him regularly.

Neither my wife nor our baby daughter did well in the United States. My wife was sick much of the time. She was weak, and she couldn't breast feed, so we gave our daughter baby formula made from cow's milk. I would work all day at the hospital and come home and help my wife, who was pregnant again. I changed the diapers and gave the baby a bottle, but my daughter cried a lot and then she developed a rash all over her skin. She was itching and miserable.

Then my son was born. His arrival was a joy, but before long he developed rectal bleeding. About that time I had acquired the first primitive colonoscope, so I was able to examine my little son and found an inflammation of the colon, or ulcerative colitis.

I was devastated. Here I was, a doctor, but I couldn't cure my beautiful young wife or relieve the suffering of my son or daughter. I hadn't learned anything in medical school that would tell me what was causing them to be sick. I consulted other doctors, the best I knew, but no one could help me. Being a skillful surgeon or giving medicine for symptoms was not enough. I wanted to know what caused disease.

In Japan I had never seen the kind of atrophic dermatitis that my daughter had, so I started investigating what in the U.S. could cause my daughter to have this. In Japan we didn't have much dairy food so I thought perhaps it was the cow's milk in her baby formula. When we took away the milk she quickly improved, and I realized she was allergic to the cow's milk. She couldn't digest it and undigested particles that were small enough to pass from her intestines into her blood were attacked by her immune system as if they were foreign invaders. The same thing turned out to be true with my son. When we stopped giving him milk his colitis disappeared.

My wife's illness was finally diagnosed as lupus. Her blood count would drop and she would become pale and anemic. She was in and out of the hospital as we struggled to save her life. She died before I knew enough to help her.

Even today I can't say what caused her lupus, but I do know that she was genetically predisposed to have an over-reactive immune system. She went to a Westernized convent school when she was growing up in Japan where they gave her lots of milk. No doubt she was allergic to milk, as her two children would later be. Exposed over and over again to a food that created an allergic reaction, her immune system must have been depleted, leaving her open to the autoimmune disease of lupus.

Because of these experiences, I began to understand how vital diet is to our health. That was over fifty years ago and in the years since, I have examined the stomachs and colons and taken the dietary history of more than 300,000 patients.

I've spent my life trying to understand the human body, health and disease. I started out focusing on disease—what caused it and how to cure it—but as I began to understand more fully how the body works as a whole system, I changed the way I treat disease. I saw that we medical professionals and our patients should spend more time understanding health than fighting disease.

We are born with the right to health; it is natural to be healthy. Once I started understanding health I began to be able to work with the body, helping it to rid itself of disease. Only the body can heal itself. As a doctor, I create a space for that healing to happen.

So I started out trying to understand disease, but eventually my research led me to what I believe is the key to health. This key is our body's own miracle enzyme.

We have over 5000 enzymes in the human body that create perhaps 25,000 different reactions. You could say that every action in our body is controlled by enzymes, but we know very little about them. I believe we create these different enzymes out of a base or source enzyme, which is more or less finite in our body. If we exhaust these source enzymes, they are not available in sufficient numbers to properly repair cells, so, over time, cancer and other degenerative diseases develop.

This, in a nutshell, is the enzyme factor.

When I help my colon cancer patients heal, I first remove the cancer from the colon, and then I put them on a very strict diet of high-enzyme, non-toxic food and water so that they have more source enzymes to use for repairing the body's cells. I do not believe in using strong drugs that defeat the immune system, because I see that the cancer in the colon did not happen as an accidental, isolated incident. The cancer in the colon is telling me the whole body's source enzyme supply is being depleted and can no longer repair the cells properly.

While I believe that we are born with a limited supply of this source enzyme and we should not deplete it with bad food, toxins, poor elimination and stress, I have come to understand something else. That something else is why I call this source enzyme a "miracle" enzyme. I have witnessed spontaneous healings and remissions of all kinds of disease. As I studied these healings further, I began to understand how such miracles can happen.

We have discovered DNA but we don't know really that much about it. There is much potential sleeping in our DNA that we don't yet understand. My research indicates that a surge of positive emotional energy, such as that arising from love, laughter, and joy, can stimulate our DNA to produce a cascade of our body's source enzyme—the miracle enzyme that acts as a bio-catalyst for repairing our cells. Joy and love can awaken a potential far beyond our current human understanding.

However, the most important thing I can tell you to live a long and healthy life is to do what makes you happy (even if that means you occasionally don't follow my other recommendations).

Play music. Make love. Have fun. Enjoy simple pleasures. Live life with passion. Remember that a happy and meaningful life is nature's way to human health. Joyful enthusiasm, rather than perfect adherence to some dietary regime, is the key to making the enzyme factor work for you.

DR. HIROMI SHINYA
June, 2007

Dr. Shinya's 7 Golden Keys for Good Health

**Use these keys to preserve your body's "Miracle Enzyme"
and enjoy a long and healthy life.**

1. A Good Diet

1. 85–90% Plant-based foods:

    a. 50% whole grains, brown rice, whole wheat pasta, barley, cereals, whole grain bread & beans including soybeans, kidney beans, garbanzo beans, lentils, pinto beans, pigeon peas, black, white & pink beans

    b. 30% green and yellow vegetables and root vegetables, including potatoes, carrots, yams and beets, and sea vegetables

    c. 5–10% fruits, seeds & nuts

2. 10–15% Animal-based proteins
(no more than 3 to 4 oz per day):

    a. Fish any type but preferably small fish as the larger fish contain mercury

    b. Poultry: chicken, turkey, duck—small amounts only

    c. Beef, lamb, veal, pork—should be limited or avoided

    d. Eggs

    e. Soy milk, soy cheese, rice milk, almond milk.

Foods to add to your diet:

1. Herbal teas
2. Seaweed tablets (kelp)
3. Brewer's yeast (good source of B complex vitamins and minerals)
4. Bee pollen and propolis
5. Enzyme supplements
6. Multi-vitamin & mineral supplements

Foods & substances to avoid or limit in your diet:

1. Dairy products such as cow's milk, cheese, yogurt, other milk products
2. Japanese green tea, Chinese tea, English tea (limit to 1–2 cups per day)
3. Coffee
4. Sweets and sugar
5. Nicotine
6. Alcohol
7. Chocolate
8. Fat and oils
9. Regular table salt (Use sea salt with trace minerals.)

Additional Dietary Recommendations:

1. Stop eating and drinking 4–5 hours before bedtime.
2. Chew every mouthful 30–50 times.
3. Do not eat between meals except for whole fruit (If hunger keeps you awake a piece of whole fruit may be eaten one hour before bedtime as it digests quickly.)
4. Eat fruits and drink juices 30–60 minutes before meals.
5. Eat whole, unrefined grains and cereals.
6. Eat more food raw or lightly steamed. Heating food over 118 degrees will kill enzymes.
7. Do not eat oxidized foods (Fruit, which has turned brown, has begun to oxidize).
8. Eat fermented foods.
9. Be disciplined with the food you eat. Remember you are what you eat.

2. Good Water

Water is essential for your health. Drink water with strong reduction power that has not been polluted with chemical substances. Drinking "good water" such as mineral water or hard water, which has much calcium and magnesium, keeps your body at an optimal alkaline pH.

- Adults should drink at least 6–10 cups of water every day.
- Drink 1–3 cups of water after waking up in the morning.
- Drink 2–3 cups of water about one hour before each meal.

3. Regular Elimination

- Start a daily habit to remove intestinal pollutants and to clean out your system regularly.
- Do not take laxatives.
- If the bowel is sluggish or to detoxify the liver, consider using a coffee enema. The coffee enema is better for colon detox and for full body detox because it does not release free radicals into the blood stream, as do some dietary detox methods.

4. Moderate Exercise

- Exercise appropriate for your age and physical condition is necessary for good health but excessive exercise can release free radicals and harm your body.
- Some good forms of exercise are walking (2.5 miles), swimming, tennis, bicycling, golf, muscle strengthening, yoga, martial arts and aerobics.

5. Adequate Rest

- Go to bed at the same time every night and get 6 to 8 hours of uninterrupted sleep.
- Do not eat or drink 4 or 5 hours before bedtime. If you are hungry or thirsty a small piece of fruit may be eaten one hour before retiring as it will digest quickly.
- Take a short nap of about 30 minutes after lunch.

6. Breathing and Meditation

- Practice meditation.
- Practice positive thinking.
- Do deep abdominal breathing 4 or 5 times per hour. The exhale should be twice as long as the inhale. This is very important as deep breaths help to rid the body of toxins and free radicals.
- Wear loose clothing that does not restrict your breath.
- Listen to your own body and be good to yourself.

7. Joy and Love

- Joy and love will boost your body's enzyme factor, sometimes in miraculous ways.
- Take time every day for an attitude of appreciation.
- Laugh.
- Sing.
- Dance.
- Live passionately and engage your life, your work, and the ones you love with your full heart.

www.ingramcontent.com/pod-product-compliance
Lightning Source LLC
Chambersburg PA
CBHW070256290326
41930CB00041B/2582